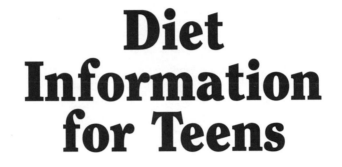

Diet Information for Teens

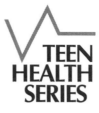

TEEN HEALTH SERIES

First Edition

Diet Information for Teens

Health Tips about Diet and Nutrition

*Including Facts about Nutrients,
Dietary Guidelines, Breakfasts, School
Lunches, Snacks, Party Food, Weight Control,
Eating Disorders, and More*

◆

Edited by Karen Bellenir

Omnigraphics

615 Griswold Street • Detroit, MI 48226

Bibliographic Note

Because this page cannot legibly accommodate all the copyright notices, the Bibliographic Note portion of the Preface constitutes an extension of the copyright notice.

Edited by Karen Bellenir

Teen Health Series

Karen Bellenir, *Managing Editor*
Joan Margeson, *Research Associate*
Dawn Matthews, *Verification Assistant*
Jenifer Swanson, *Research Associate*

Omnigraphics, Inc.

Matthew P. Barbour, *Vice President, Operations*
Laurie Lanzen Harris, *Vice President, Editorial Director*
Kevin Hayes, *Production Coordinator*
Thomas J. Murphy, *Vice President, Finance and Comptroller*
Peter E. Ruffner, *Senior Vice President*
Jane J. Steele, *Marketing Consultant*

Frederick G. Ruffner, Jr., *Publisher*

Library of Congress Cataloging-in-Publication Data

Diet information for teens : health tips about diet and nutrition, including facts about nutrients, dietary guidelines, breakfasts, school lunches, snacks, party foods, weight control, eating disorders, and more / edited by Karen Bellenir.
    p. cm -- (Teen health series)
  Includes bibliographical references and index.
  ISBN 0-7808-0441-4
    1. Teenagers--Nutrition. 2. Teenagers--Health and hygiene. 3. Diet. 4. Health. I. Bellenir, Karen. II. Series.

RJ235 .D546 2000
613.2'0835--dc21

                      00-049213

∞

Table of Contents

Part 3: Meal Planning

Part 4: Weight Control

Part 5: Eating Disorders

Part 6: If You Need More Information

Preface

About This Book

During the teen years, boys and girls complete their final major growth spurt before adulthood. For girls, these finishing touches add some fat padding. Boys add muscle and increase their volume of blood. These changes often encourage girls to diet unnecessarily to stay slim, while boys may overeat to satisfy their appetites. Neither practice produces good results, and both can lead to health problems in future years.

This book provides information about making good food choices, following nutrition guidelines, and coping with special dietary needs. It offers tips for planning breakfasts, lunches, dinners, and snacks. It describes the best and worst ways to try to loose weight, and it provides help for people who want to gain weight. A special section on eating disorders describes anorexia nervosa, bulimia nervosa, and binge eating disorder. At the end of this book, readers will find a directory of other resources, a list of additional reading materials, and a bibliography of cookbooks.

How To Use This Book

This book is divided into parts and chapters. Parts focus on broad areas of interest. Chapters are devoted to single topics within a part.

Part I: Food Fundamentals describes basic principles of good nutrition. It provides facts about vitamins and minerals, dietary supplements, fats, and fiber. A chapter on the special concerns of people with food allergies and intolerances is also included. If you are looking for general information about how food fuels your body, try the chapters in this part.

Part II: Dietary Choices offers guidelines for healthy eating. It includes information about using the food guide pyramid, reading food labels, and evaluating school lunches. It offers tips on making good food and beverage choices in a variety of circumstances, such as eating out, battling the "munchies," and preparing for sports events. If you are looking for guidance about the foods you choose to eat, the chapters in this part can help steer you in the right direction.

Part III: Meal Planning provides the information you need to help put your food choices into action. It offers information on planning great menus for breakfast, lunch, dinner, and even snacks. A chapter on food safety explains how to keep foodborne illnesses from spoiling an otherwise healthy meal. If you are ready to roll up your sleeves and get to work in the kitchen, this part is for you.

Part IV: Weight Control includes information for people who want to loose or gain weight. It describes the principles of good weight loss programs and offers cautions about dietary practices that may be a threat to good health. If you want to shed some pounds—or if you need to gain a few—the chapters in this part will help as you begin working toward your goal.

Part V: Eating Disorders describes the signs, symptoms, and need for treatment for three major eating disorders: anorexia nervosa, bulimia nervosa, and binge eating disorder. When left untreated, eating disorders can lead to serious health problems and even death. If you are worried about a friend's eating habits, or if you think you may have a problem, the chapters in this part will give you background information so that you can seek professional help.

Part VI: If You Need More Information provides a directory of resources, a list of additional reading materials, and a bibliography of cookbooks that may be of special interest to teens.

Bibliographic Note

This volume contains documents and excerpts from publications issued by the following government agencies: National Institute of Allergy and Infectious Diseases (NIAID), National Institute of Dental and Craniofacial

Research (NIDCR), National Institute of Diabetes and Digestive and Kidney Diseases (NIDDK), U.S. Department of Agriculture (USDA), U.S. Federal Trade Commission (FTC), and the U.S. Food and Drug Administration (FDA).

In addition, this volume contains copyrighted articles produced by Liz Applegate, Ph.D.; Center for Science in the Public Interest; Clinical Reference Systems; InteliHealth; Iowa State University; Nemours Foundation; and the University of Delaware, Delaware Cooperative Extension. Copyrighted articles from the following periodicals are also included: *Consumer's Research Magazine*; *Current Health 2* (Weekly Reader Corp.); and *Tufts University Diet and Nutrition Letter*.

Full citation information is provided on the first page of each chapter. Every effort has been made to secure all necessary rights to reprint the copyrighted material. If any omissions have been made, please contact Omnigraphics to make corrections for future editions.

Acknowledgements

In addition to the organizations listed above, special thanks are due to researchers Jenifer Swanson and Joan Margeson, verification assistant Dawn Matthews, permissions specialist Maria Franklin, and editorial assistant Buffy Bellenir.

Note From The Editor

This book is part of Omnigraphics' *Teen Health Series*. The series provides basic information about a broad range of medical concerns. It is not intended to serve as a tool for diagnosing illness, in prescribing treatments, or as a substitute for the physician/patient relationship. All persons concerned about medical symptoms or the possibility of disease are encouraged to seek professional care from an appropriate health care provider.

The *Teen Health Series*, a specially focused set of volumes within Omnigraphics' *Health Reference Series*, was developed at the request of librarians serving today's young adults. Each volume deals comprehensively with a topic selected according to the needs and interests of people in middle school and high school. If there is a subject you would like to see addressed in a future volume of the *Teen Health Series*, please write to:

Editor, *Teen Health Series*
Omnigraphics, Inc.
615 Griswold Street
Detroit, MI 48226

Our Advisory Board

The *Teen Health Series* is reviewed by an Advisory Board comprised of librarians from public, academic, and medical libraries. We would like to thank the following board members for providing guidance to the development of this series:

Dr. Lynda Baker
Associate Professor of Library and Information Science
Wayne State University, Detroit, MI

Nancy Bulgarelli
William Beaumont Hospital Library
Royal Oak, MI

Karen Imarasio
Bloomfield Township Public Library
Bloomfield Township, MI

Karen Morgan
Mardigian Library, University of Michigan-Dearborn
Dearborn, MI

Rosemary Orlando
St. Clair Shores Public Library
St. Clair Shores, MI

Part 1

Food Fundamentals

Chapter 1

Good News About Good Nutrition

You've heard it all before. For as long as you can remember, your parents, your teachers, perhaps even your doctor, have been telling you to eat your vegetables, limit sweets, drink your milk.

Now, in your teen years, this advice takes on new meaning for a lot of very different reasons: How can you gain weight to put on muscle instead of fat? What's a healthy weight for you? How can you squeeze in a good, quick meal after school and before you have to be at your part-time job? All good questions, and because of the enormous changes that are going on in your body, the way you decide to deal with your nutrition needs now can make a big difference not only in how you feel today, but also in your well-being in years to come.

If you are between 15 and 18, you're completing your final major growth spurt, and are in the process of putting on nature's finishing touches for adulthood. For girls, the finishing touch means adding some fat padding. For boys, it means adding muscle and increasing the volume of blood. These changes often encourage girls to diet unnecessarily to stay slim, while boys may overeat to satisfy their appetites. Both can lead to health problems down the road, and, incidentally, probably will not do the job you want right now.

About This Chapter: The text in this chapter is from "On the Teen Scene: Good News About Good Nutrition," by Judith E. Foulke, an article that oginally appeared in the April 1992 *FDA Consumer*. This version is from a reprint of that article, Publication No. (FDA) 99-2257; it contains revisions made in April 1995, December 1996, and January 1999.

So what is the right approach to healthy eating?

A good start is to eat a variety of foods, as suggested in the *Dietary Guidelines for Americans*, published by the U.S. Departments of Agriculture and Health and Human Services. Get the many nutrients your body needs by choosing a variety of foods from each of these groups:

- vegetables
- fruits
- breads, cereals, rice, and pasta

- milk, yogurt, and cheese
- meat, poultry, fish, dried beans and peas, eggs, and nuts

What's So Junky About 'Junk' Food?

The pace for teens is fast and getting faster. Added to pressures from school to prepare for college or a job, many teens take part in sports and work part-time. This often means eating on the run. Stack that on top of the snack foods you eat on dates or when you get together with friends, and the balance of your nutrients can get way out of kilter.

Many snacks, such as potato chips, fast-food cheeseburgers, and fries, have high levels of fat, sugar, or salt—ingredients that are usually best limited to a small portion of your diet. Healthy eating doesn't mean that you can't have your favorite foods, but the *Dietary Guidelines* advise you to be selective and limit the total fat, saturated fat, cholesterol, and sodium you eat. Our main source of saturated fat comes from animal products and hydrogenated vegetable oils, with tropical oils—coconut and palm—providing smaller amounts. Only animal fat provides cholesterol. Sodium mostly comes from salt added to foods during processing, home preparation, or at the table.

Fats are our most concentrated source of energy. Scientists know that eating too much fat, especially saturated fat and cholesterol, increases blood cholesterol levels, and therefore increases your risk of heart disease. Too much fat also may lead to overweight and increase your risk of some cancers.

Dietitians recommend that no more than 30 percent of your calories come from fats, and not more than 10 percent of these calories should be from saturated fat. Choose lean meats, fish, poultry without skin, and low-fat dairy

✎ Weird Words

<u>Anorexia Nervosa:</u> An eating disorder with a loss of appetite for food, characterized by a fear of gaining weight or becoming fat.

<u>Bulimia Nervosa:</u> An earing disorder characterized by eating large amounts of food in short time periods. One type includes self-induced vomiting or the abuse of laxatives to control weight; another type includes strict dieting, fasting, or excessive exercising.

<u>Calorie:</u> Calories measure the energy your body gets from food. Your body needs calories as "fuel" to perform all of its functions such as breathing, circulating the blood, and physical activity.

<u>Cholesterol:</u> A fat-like substance in the body. The body makes and needs some cholesterol, which also comes from foods such as butter and egg yolks. Too much may cause a disease that slows or stops blood flow.

<u>Dehydration:</u> When the body loses too much water.

<u>Hydrogenated Fat:</u> A fat that has been chemically altered by the addition of hydrogen atoms to convert it to a semi-solid form such as margarine or shortening.

<u>Osteoporosis:</u> A disease that causes bones to become thin and brittle.

products whenever you can. When you eat out, particularly at fast-food restaurants, look for broiled or baked rather than fried foods. Try the salad bars more often, but pass up creamy items and limit the amount of salad dressing you use to keep down the fat and calories. Look for milk-based high-calcium foods with reduced fat.

Spare The Sugar And Salt

Most people like the taste of table sugar. But did you know that other sweeteners are sometimes "hidden" in foods? There are sugars in honey, dried fruits, concentrated fruit juices, and ingredients such as corn syrup that are added to soft drinks, cookies, and many other processed foods. You can see what sugars are in packaged foods by looking at the ingredient list.

If you are a very active teen with high-energy needs, sweets can be an additional source of calories. But keep in mind that they contain only limited nutrients and that both sugars and starches can contribute to tooth decay.

A moderate amount of sodium in your diet is necessary, because sodium, along with potassium, maintains the water balance in your body. But for some people, too much sodium can be a factor in high blood pressure. Since processed foods often contain large amounts of sodium, it's wise to use salt sparingly when cooking or at the table—and to avoid overeating salty snacks like pretzels and chips.

When you exercise heavily and sweat profusely, you can deplete your sodium reserve, unbalance your body chemistry, and possibly become dehydrated. In extreme cases of profuse sweating, such as during training or competition, a dilute glucose-electrolyte drink may become necessary, but always with an abundance of water to make up for sweat losses.

What's All This About Fiber?

Whole-grain breads and cereals, dried beans and peas, vegetables, and fruits contain various types of dietary fiber essential for proper bowel function. Eating plenty of these fiber-rich foods may reduce your risk of cancer and heart disease.

The benefits from a high-fiber diet may be related to the foods themselves and not to fiber alone. For this reason, it's best to get fiber from foods rather than from the fiber supplements you can purchase in a store.

Be Aware Of Alcohol

Alcoholic beverages deserve special mention. Drinking them risks good health and can cause other serious problems for teens. And although it is illegal for teens to buy alcoholic beverages, a 1994 survey conducted by the Department of Health and Human Services shows that 31 percent of high-school seniors and 20 percent of juniors reported being drunk in the past 30 days.

♣ **It's A Fact!!**

Alcoholic beverages contain calories but few if any nutrients.

Teens who drink risk impaired judgment in their social relationships and endanger their own and others' lives if they drive after drinking. According to the U.S. Department of Transportation, in 1996, 37 percent of fatal crashes involving 15- to 20-year-old drivers were alcohol-related.

Alcoholic beverages contain calories but few if any nutrients. Drinking heavily can lead to poor nutrition if alcoholic beverages replace foods with needed nutrients, and alcoholism is not unknown among teenagers.

What About Vegetarians?

There are many types of vegetarian diets, but the two most common are the lacto-ovo, which includes eggs and milk products but not meat, and vegan, which eliminates all forms of animal products. Teens who are lacto-ovo vegetarians can usually get enough nutrients in their diets.

Vegan vegetarians are vulnerable to deficiencies of several nutrients, particularly vitamins D and B_{12}, calcium, iron, zinc, and perhaps other trace elements. Like all essential nutrients, these vitamins and minerals are required to maintain proper growth.

If it is important to you to be a vegetarian, it is easier to achieve good nutrition with the lacto-ovo form. A dietitian (or your school nurse) can help you plan a vegetarian diet that provides you with the nutrients you need for growth and development during the teen years.

Iron And Calcium

The need for iron for both boys and girls increases between the ages of 11 and 18. The National Academy of Sciences recommends teenage boys get 12 milligrams of iron a day, mostly to sustain their rapidly enlarging body mass. For girls, the recommended daily requirement is 15 milligrams to offset menstrual losses that begin during this time.

It's important to plan how to get adequate iron in your diet. Iron from meat, poultry, and fish is better absorbed by your body than the iron from plant sources. However, the absorption of iron from plants is improved by eating fruit or drinking juice that contains vitamin C with the iron-rich food.

☞ Remember!!

Dietary Guidelines For All Americans

What should Americans eat to stay healthy? These guidelines, published by the U.S. Departments of Agriculture and Health and Human Services, reflect recommendations of nutrition authorities who agree that enough is known about the effect of diet on health to encourage certain dietary practices. The guidelines are:

- Eat a variety of foods.

- Balance the food you eat with physical activity—maintain a healthy weight.

- Choose a diet with plenty of grain products, vegetables, and fruits.

- Choose a diet low in fat, saturated fat, and cholesterol.

- Choose a diet moderate in sugars.

- Choose a diet moderate in salt and sodium.

- Children and adolescents should not drink alcoholic beverages.

The Dietary Guidelines suggest at least the following number of servings from each of these food groups:

- Vegetables: 3-5 servings

- Fruits: 2-4 servings

- Breads, cereals, rice, and pasta: 6-11 servings

- Milk, yogurt, and cheese: 2-3 servings, however teenagers should have three or more servings daily of foods rich in calcium.

- Meats, poultry, fish, dried beans and peas, eggs, and nuts: 2-3 servings

Teens need extra calcium to store up an optimal amount of bone (called "peak" bone mass). The richest sources of calcium are milk and other dairy products. Building optimal bone mass through a balanced diet, including adequate calcium, may help delay the onset or limit your chances of developing osteoporosis later in life. Osteoporosis is a disease in which reduced bone mass causes bones to break easily. It occurs in both men and women, but is more common among older women.

What's A Healthy Weight?

Some teens have a difficult time projecting a healthy weight for themselves. Girls especially may think they need to be thinner than they are, or should be. Extraordinary concern or obsession for thinness leads some teens to the eating disorders of anorexia nervosa (dieting to starvation) or bulimia (overeating and then vomiting).

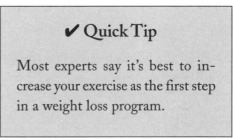

✔ Quick Tip

Most experts say it's best to increase your exercise as the first step in a weight loss program.

If you're concerned about your weight, it's important to talk to a health professional such as your family doctor or the school nurse. That person can help you decide whether you do need to lose weight and, if so, the best way to achieve and maintain a weight that is healthy for you.

If health professionals recommend that you need to lose weight, most experts say it's best to increase your exercise as the first step. Often that's all teens need to do for weight control because they're rapidly growing. If eating less is also necessary, it is best to continue eating a variety of foods while cutting down on fats and sugars.

Losing weight quickly on a very low-calorie diet is never a good idea for anyone. And if you're into sports, you should be aware that it could affect your athletic performance. Under no circumstances should you drink less fluid to lose weight. A steady loss of a pound or so a week until you reach your goal is generally safe, and you're more likely to be able to maintain your weight loss.

Skipping meals to lose weight is another poor idea. You're likely to over-eat at the next meal just because you're so hungry. And surveys show that people who skip breakfast or other meals tend to have poorer nutrition than those who don't.

Help For Healthy Eating

The food label can help nutrition-conscious people make wise food choices. This can be important to teens who sometimes shop not only for themselves but also for the whole family.

The Nutrition Labeling and Education Act of 1990, enforced by FDA, requires almost all food products to be labeled with the nutritive values they contain per serving. Serving sizes now are more uniform across all product lines, so that you can more easily compare the nutritional values of similar foods; for example, ice cream and frozen yogurt. And the serving sizes are closer to amounts people really eat.

Also, the government has set strict definitions for claims like "low fat" and "light," so when you see them, you can believe them.

FDA now allows food labels to carry claims about the relationship between a food or nutrient and a disease or health-related condition; for example, calcium and a reduced risk of osteoporosis, a bone disease; and sodium and an increased risk of high blood pressure. So far, FDA has approved 10 claims, which are supported by significant scientific evidence.

Thanks to the growing scientific knowledge about diet and health relationships, healthy eating is more socially "in" than ever before. Eating a healthy diet is not difficult with knowledge of a few of the basics and can help you excel on the playing field, in school, and in your social life.

Chapter 2

What You Need To Know About Vitamins And Minerals

Fat-Soluble Vitamins

Vitamin A

- *Good to know:* Also called retinol or retinoic acid. Humans convert carotenes from plant foods into vitamin A in the body.

- *Recommendations:*

  Men ages 11–51+, 1000 micrograms RE/day (equivalent to about 5000 IU)

  Women ages 11–51+, 800 micrograms RE/day (equivalent to about 4000 IU)

  Note: RE = retinol equivalent, the standard measure for vitamin A.

- *Benefits:* Important for good vision, especially at night. Also affects immunity, reproduction, and the growth and maintenance of cells of the skin, gastrointestinal tract, and other mucus membranes.

- *Food sources:* Fortified milk, eggs, liver, cheese, leafy green vegetables (such as spinach, kale, turnip greens, collards, and Romaine lettuce), broccoli, dark orange fruits and vegetables (such as apricots, carrots, pumpkin, sweet potatoes, papaya, mango, and cantaloupe), red bell pepper.

About This Chapter: Text in this chapter is from "Vitamins and Minerals: A to Z Glossary," at www.intelihealth.com, © 1999 InteliHealth Inc.; reprinted with permission.

- Day's supply in: ½ cup sweet potatoes (2800 micrograms [mcg]), OR one carrot (2000 mcg), OR 1 oz fortified cornflakes (635 mcg) PLUS 1 cup milk (150 mcg) PLUS 1 cup raw spinach (375 mcg).

- *Watch out:* Taking high-dose supplements (daily dose over 15,000 micrograms RE, or about 75,000 IU) can cause toxicity, which can result in bone fractures; joint pain; headaches; skin that is dry, itchy or peeling; brittle nails; hair loss; nausea and vomiting; diarrhea; fatigue; blurred vision; liver failure; hemorrhages.

Vitamin D

- *Good to know:* The body can make vitamin D on its own, provided it gets enough sunlight. By exposing face, hands, and forearms for between 5 and 30 minutes two or three times per week, most people can manufacture all the vitamin D they need. Sunscreen blocks the type of rays needed to produce vitamin D.

- *Recommendations:*
    Ages 11–24, 10 micrograms/day (equivalent to about 400 IU)
    Ages 25–50, 5 micrograms/day (equivalent to about 200 IU)

✎ Weird Words

Fat-Soluble Vitamins: Vitamins A, D, E, and K are fat-soluble, meaning that they dissolve in fat and are carried by fat molecules throughout the body. If we had no fat in our diets, we would be unable to reap the benefits of these vitamins. These vitamins also can be stored in body fat, so taking supplements of fat-soluble vitamins—especially vitamin A or vitamin D—is risky unless prescribed by a doctor, since the stored excess can build up to dangerous levels.

Water-Soluble Vitamins: The B-vitamins and vitamin C are water-soluble, which means that they dissolve in water and are carried throughout the body in the bloodstream. These vitamins are not stored in the body. After the body uses what it needs, any excess is excreted in urine.

Minerals: Like vitamins, minerals are essential nutrients required to help the body function properly.

Ages 51–70, 10 micrograms/day (equivalent to about 400 IU)
Ages 71+, 15 micrograms/day (equivalent to about 600 IU)
Note: IU = International Unit.

- *Benefits:* Increases absorption of calcium and phosphorus, which leads to stronger bones and teeth.

- *Food sources:* Fish liver oils, fatty fish, fortified milk, cheese, egg yolk, and fortified cereals. Sunlight helps the body create its own vitamin D.

- *Day's supply in:* 2 cups milk (200 IU), OR 1 cup milk (100 IU) PLUS 1 cup cornflakes (40 IU) PLUS 1 egg (25 IU) PLUS 1 tsp margarine (20 IU) PLUS 3 ounces salmon with bones (10 IU).

- *Watch out:* Since vitamin D is absorbed in the small intestines, people with diseases that prevent proper absorption—such as liver disease, cystic fibrosis, Whipple's disease, and sprue—may develop vitamin D deficiency. Vitamin D production plateaus after a short amount of time in the sun. More exposure won't produce extra vitamin D, just skin damage. Excess vitamin D from supplements (greater than 50 micrograms or 2000 IU per day) can result in kidney damage, kidney stones, weakened bones and muscles, and possibly death.

Vitamin E

- *Good to know:* Also called alpha-tocopherol, tocopherol, or tocotrienol. Alpha-tocopherol is the most biologically active form.

- *Recommendations:*
     Men ages 11–51+, 10 milligrams/day (equivalent to about 30 IU)
     Women ages 11–51+, 8 milligrams/day (equivalent to about 24 IU)

- *Benefits:* Acts as an antioxidant, reducing risks of cancer and heart disease; contributes to good immunity.

- *Food sources:* Vegetable oils, wheat germ, whole-grain products, nuts, egg yolks, green leafy vegetables.

- *Day's supply in:* 1 ounce wheat germ (5 mg) PLUS 1 egg (0.5 mg) PLUS 1 ounce toasted almonds (4.5 mg).

- *Watch out:* No warnings.

Vitamin K

- *Good to know:* Also called menadione, menaquinone, or phylloquinone. Vitamin K is made in the body by normal intestinal bacteria, then absorbed for use.

- *Recommendations:*

  Men ages 15–18, 70 micrograms/day
  Men ages 19–24, 70 micrograms/day
  Men ages 25+, 80 micrograms/day
  Women ages 15–18, 55 micrograms/day
  Women ages 19–24, 60 micrograms/day
  Women ages 25+, 65 micrograms/day

- *Benefits:* Makes proteins that allow the blood to clot.

- *Food sources:* Liver, cabbage, broccoli, green leafy vegetables (such as spinach, kale, collard, and turnip greens), milk, eggs, citrus fruits.

- *Day's supply in:* 1 cup raw spinach (145 mcg), OR half cup raw broccoli (60 mcg) PLUS 1 egg (25 mcg).

- *Watch out:* Too much vitamin K can interfere with anti-clotting medications such as warfarin (Coumadin).

Water-Soluble Vitamins

Thiamin

- *Good to know:* Also called vitamin B_1, vitamin F, thiamine.

- *Recommendations:*

  Men ages 14–70+, 1.2 milligrams/day
  Women ages 14–18, 1.0 milligrams/day
  Women ages 19–70+, 1.1 milligrams/day

- *Benefits:* Important for producing energy from carbohydrates, and for proper nerve function.

- *Food sources:* Pork, liver, legumes, nuts, whole grain or enriched breads and cereals.

- *Day's supply in:* 1 broiled pork chop (0.66 mg) PLUS 1.25 cups corn flakes (0.36 mg) OR 1 baked potato with skin (0.24 mg) PLUS ½ cup lentils (0.17 mg) PLUS 1 cup raisin bran (0.60 mg).

- *Watch out:* Deficiency is becoming more common among the homeless and malnourished people, and can result in edema and heart arrhythmias.

Riboflavin

- *Good to know:* Also called vitamin B$_2$.

- *Recommendations:*

    Men ages 14–70+, 1.3 milligrams/day
    Women ages 14–18, 1.0 milligrams/day
    Ages 71+, 15 micrograms/day (equivalent to about 600 IU)

- *Benefits:* Contributes to energy production.

- *Food sources:* Lean meats, yogurt, milk, cheese, egg, broccoli, whole grain or enriched breads and cereals.

- *Day's supply in:* 1 cup raisin bran cereal (0.7 mg) PLUS 1 cup milk (0.34 mg) PLUS 1 egg (0.25 mg) OR one small extra-lean hamburger (0.36 mg) PLUS 1 cup plain yogurt (0.49 mg) PLUS ½ cup fresh cooked spinach (0.21) PLUS 1 cup cottage cheese (0.36 mg).

- *Watch out:* Light can destroy riboflavin, so purchase milk in opaque containers.

Niacin

- *Good to know:* Also called nicotinic acid, nicotinamide, vitamin B$_3$. The human body can make niacin from the amino acid tryptophan, so any food high in tryptophan, such as turkey, will contribute to niacin intake.

- *Recommendations:*

    Men ages 14–70+, 16 milligrams NE/day
    Women ages 14–70+, 14 milligrams NE/day
    Note: NE = niacin equivalent

- *Benefits:* Contributes to energy production. Important for health of skin, digestive tract, and nervous system.

- *Food sources:* Protein-rich foods, including milk, eggs, meat, poultry, fish, nuts, and enriched cereals and grain products.

- *Day's supply in:* One small extra-lean hamburger (6.63 mg) PLUS ½ cup Grape Nuts cereal (9.98 mg) OR 1 cup rice (2 mg) PLUS 4 ounces broiled salmon (7.5 mg) PLUS 1 tablespoon peanut butter (4.22 mg) PLUS 1 bagel (3.1 mg).

- *Watch out:* In high doses, nicotinic acid can cause dilation of blood vessels and a potentially painful tingling called a "niacin flush." High doses of niacin can cause diarrhea, nausea, and vomiting. In the long-term, liver damage may result.

Biotin

- *Good to know:* Because biotin is contained in many foods and requirements are so small, virtually no one needs to worry about deficiency.

- *Recommendations:*
    > Ages 14–18, 25 micrograms/day
    > Ages 19–70+, 30 micrograms/day

- *Benefits:* Contributes to energy production and metabolism of proteins, fats, and carbohydrates.

- *Food sources:* Found in many foods, especially liver, egg yolks, and cereal.

- *Day's supply in:* Any combination of healthy foods.

- *Watch out:* Although deficiency is rare, it can be caused by eating high quantities of raw egg whites, which bind biotin and make it unavailable to the body.

Pantothenic Acid

- *Good to know:* Deficiencies are rare among people with a healthy diet.

- *Recommendations:*
    > Ages 14–70+, 5 milligrams/day

- *Benefits:* Contributes to energy production

- *Food sources:* Found in many foods, especially meat, poultry, fish, egg yolk, legumes, and cereals.

- *Day's supply in:* Any combination of healthy foods.

- *Watch out:* No warnings.

Vitamin B$_6$

- *Good to know:* Also called pyridoxine.

- *Recommendations:*
    Men ages 14–50, 1.3 milligrams/day
    Men ages 51–70+, 1.7 milligrams/day
    Women ages 14–18, 1.2 milligrams/day
    Women ages 19–50, 1.3 milligrams/day
    Women ages 51–70+, 1.5 milligrams/day

- *Benefits:* Helps the body make red blood cells, converts tryptophan to niacin, and contributes to immunity and nervous system function. Used in metabolism of proteins and fats.

- *Food sources:* Meats, fish, poultry, legumes, leafy green vegetables, potatoes, bananas, fortified cereals.

- *Day's supply in:* 1 chicken breast (1.0 mg) PLUS ½ cup cooked spinach (0.22 mg) PLUS 1 cup brown rice (0.28 mg), OR 1 baked potato with skin (0.69 mg) PLUS 1 banana (0.66) PLUS 4 oz lean sirloin (0.51 mg).

- *Watch out:* High-dose vitamin B$_6$ supplements have been recommended to help PMS, carpal tunnel syndrome, and sleep disorders. However, taking very high doses for months or years can cause permanent nerve damage. Recommended upper limit is 100 milligrams per day for adults.

Folate

- *Good to know:* Also called folic acid or folacin.

- *Recommendations:*
    Ages 14–70+, 400 micrograms/day

- *Benefits:* Critical for all cell functions, since folate helps make DNA and RNA. May protect against heart disease by lowering homocysteine levels. In pregnant women, lowers risk of neural tube defects in the baby.

- *Food sources:* Leafy green vegetables, especially spinach and turnip greens, legumes, broccoli, asparagus, oranges, and fortified cereals.

- *Day's supply in:* 6 asparagus spears (131 mcg) PLUS 1 cup orange juice from concentrate (109 mcg) PLUS ½ cup lentils (178 mcg) PLUS 2 slices whole wheat bread (28 mcg) OR 1 cup Total cereal (465 mcg).

- *Watch out:* To prevent spina bifida and other neural tube disorders in their babies, all pregnant women—and women who have the potential to become pregnant—should be on folate supplements. For all adults, too little folate can result in anemia.

Vitamin B$_{12}$

- *Good to know:* Also called cobalamin. Although vitamin B$_{12}$ injections have been rumored to increase energy, there's no scientific evidence that this is true.

- *Recommendations:*

  Ages 14–70+, 2.4 micrograms/day

- *Benefits:* Important for proper nerve function. Works with folate, converting it to an active form. Helps make red blood cells, and helps metabolize proteins and fats.

- *Food sources:* Only found in animal foods, such as meats, fish, poultry, milk, cheese, and eggs; or in fortified cereals.

- *Day's supply in:* 1 chicken breast (0.6 mcg) PLUS 1 hard-boiled egg (0.55 mcg) PLUS 1 cup plain low-fat yogurt (1.37 mcg) OR 1 cup milk (0.92 mcg) PLUS 1 cup raisin bran (1.64 mcg).

- *Watch out:* Vegetarians, especially vegans who eat no animal foods, need to look for fortified sources, such as fortified soy milk, or supplements of vitamin B$_{12}$. The elderly often have difficulty absorbing vitamin B$_{12}$, and can easily develop deficiencies. Deficiency may result in anemia, nerve damage, and hypersensitive skin.

Vitamin C

- *Good to know:* Also called ascorbic acid. Cigarette smoke depletes vitamin C, so smokers need 100 milligrams per day.

- *Recommendations:*

  Ages 15–51+, 60 milligrams/day

- *Benefits:* Important for immune function. Acts as an antioxidant to keep the body healthy. Strengthens blood vessels and capillary walls, makes collagen and connective tissue that hold muscles and bones together, helps form scar tissue, keeps gums healthy, and helps the body absorb iron from foods.

- *Food sources:* Many fruits and vegetables, especially citrus fruits, dark green vegetables, strawberries, papaya, cantaloupe, peppers, broccoli, potatoes, and tomatoes.

- *Day's supply in:* 1 cup grapefruit juice (72 mg) OR 1 kiwi fruit (74 mg) OR 1 cup chopped broccoli (116 mg) OR 1 baked potato with skin (26 mg) PLUS 1 cup tomato juice (45 mg).

- *Watch out:* Very high doses of vitamin C supplements (over 1000 milligrams) can cause diarrhea and may cause kidney stones.

Minerals

Calcium

- *Good to know:* Calcium is believed to help prevent osteoporosis and colon cancer.

- *Recommendations:*
    Ages 11–24, 1200 milligrams/day
    Ages 25–51+, 800 milligrams/day

- *Benefits:* Critical for strengthening bones and teeth. Necessary for proper nervous system and immune function, assists in muscle contraction, blood clotting, and blood pressure.

- *Food sources:* Dairy products, including milk, yogurt, and cheese, fish with bones (such as sardines or salmon), tofu, legumes, broccoli, kale, cabbage, calcium-fortified orange juice.

- *Day's supply in:* 1 cup of milk (300 mg) PLUS 1 cup chopped broccoli (72 mg) PLUS 1 cup navy beans (127 mg) PLUS 1 cup plain yogurt (447 mg) PLUS 4 ounces canned pink salmon (242 mg).

- *Watch out:* Most people, especially women, find it difficult to get adequate amounts of calcium from diet alone. Many doctors recommend a supplement of 1000 milligrams per day.

Chloride

- *Good to know:* The greatest source of chloride in the diet is table salt, or sodium chloride.

- *Recommendations:*

    Adult minimum: 750 milligrams/day.

- *Benefits:* Important for fluid balance in the body. Also important for digestion, since it is a component of hydrochloric acid found in the stomach.

- *Food sources:* Table salt, soy sauce, processed foods.

- *Day's supply in:* The recommended minimum amount is satisfied by a mere quarter-teaspoon of table salt.

- *Watch out:* No supplementation is necessary unless recommended by a physician. Too much table salt increases the risk of hypertension in susceptible individuals.

Chromium

- *Good to know:* The dietary supplement chromium picolinate has been suggested to help burn fat and build muscle, but no scientific research has supported these claims.

- *Recommendations:* Safe and adequate amounts for everyone over age 7, 50–200 micrograms/day.

- *Benefits:* Works with insulin to help cells use glucose.

- *Food sources:* Unrefined whole grain products, liver, brewer's yeast, nuts, cheese, meats.

- *Day's supply in:* 1 ounce American cheese (48 mcg) OR 1 cup cooked peas (60 mcg) OR 2 eggs (26 mcg each).

- *Watch out:* Because most people in the U.S. eat a diet of refined foods, many people don't get even the minimal amount of chromium in their diets. Deficiency symptoms resemble diabetes because the body is unable to use insulin normally. Symptoms may include fatigue, increased thirst and urination, and extreme hunger.

Copper

- *Good to know:* Chocolate contains moderate amounts of copper. People with copper pipes get significant amounts of copper in their drinking water.

- *Recommendations:* Safe and adequate amounts for adults: 1.5–3.0 milligrams/day.

- *Benefits:* Helps make red blood cells, is part of several body enzymes, and is important for the absorption of iron.

- *Food sources:* Shellfish, nuts, seeds, legumes, whole grain products, liver, meats.

- *Day's supply in:* 1 Alaska King crab leg (1.57 mg) OR ½ cup lentils (0.25 mg) PLUS 1 cup raisin bran (0.25 mg) PLUS ½ cup roasted almonds (0.96 mg).

- *Watch out:* Copper can be depleted if too much zinc (supplements of 50 milligrams per day for a long period of time) is taken.

Fluoride

- *Good to know:* About half of all U.S. residents drink fluoridated water.

- *Recommendations:*

  Safe and adequate amounts for children ages 7–18: 1.5–2.5 milligrams/day

  Safe and adequate amounts for adults: 1.5–4.0 milligrams/day

- *Benefits:* Helps form bones and teeth, and helps make teeth decay-resistant.

- *Food sources:* Fluoridated drinking water, seafood, tea.

- *Day's supply in:* Usually attained in drinking water or through supplements.

- *Watch out:* Fluoridated water has helped reduce the amount of tooth decay among children in the U.S. But more is not necessarily better. People who get too much fluoride from a variety of sources can have permanently discolored teeth. Don't take fluoride supplements without consulting a local physician or dentist.

Iodine

- *Good to know:* Iodine is found in the soil near coastal areas, so vegetables grown near salt water will also contain iodine.

- *Recommendations:*

    Ages 11–51+, 150 micrograms/day

- *Benefits:* Regulates growth and metabolic rate as a component of thyroid hormones.

- *Food sources:* Iodized table salt, salt water fish.

- *Day's supply in:* Normally attained through iodized salt or vegetables grown in iodine-rich soil.

- *Watch out:* Iodine deficiency can result in goiter, the enlargement of the thyroid gland. Goiter is rare in the U.S.

Iron

- *Good to know:* Iron from foods is absorbed better if you also eat foods rich in vitamin C.

- *Recommendations:*

    Men ages 11–18, 12 milligrams/day
    Men ages 19–51+, 10 milligrams/day
    Women ages 11–50, 15 milligrams/day
    Women ages 51+, 10 milligrams/day

- *Benefits:* Important part of red blood cells.

- *Food sources:* Red meat, fish, poultry, eggs, legumes, fortified cereals.

- *Day's supply in:* 1 small extra-lean hamburger (3.14 mg) PLUS 1 cup dry roasted mixed nuts (5.07 mg) PLUS 1 egg (0.72 mg) PLUS ½ cup tofu (6.65 mg) OR 1 cup Kellogg's raisin bran (22.2 mg).

- *Watch out:* Iron deficiency is common throughout the world. Women are especially at risk, since they lose iron in menstrual blood. Deficiency can lead anemia, with symptoms of fatigue, weakness and ill health. Too much iron may increase the risk of heart disease in men.

Magnesium

- *Good to know:* Chocolate and cocoa are good sources of magnesium.

- *Recommendations:*

    Men ages 14–18, 410 milligrams/day
    Men ages 19–30, 400 milligrams/day
    Men ages 31–70+, 420 milligrams/day
    Women ages 14–18, 360 milligrams/day
    Women ages 19–30, 310 milligrams/day
    Women ages 31–70+, 320 milligrams/day

- *Benefits:* Part of enzymes in the body, helps build bones, teeth, and proteins, important for proper function of nerves, muscles, and immune system.

- *Food sources:* Legumes, nuts, whole grain foods, green vegetables, seafood. Day's supply in:1 cup navy beans (107 mg) PLUS 4 ounces halibut (121 mg) PLUS 1 cup brown rice (84 mg) PLUS 1 cup raisins (48 mg) PLUS ½ cup cooked spinach (65 mg).

- *Watch out:* Magnesium deficiency is rare, but people with diabetes, people who are chronically on diuretics, and chronic alcoholics are at much greater risk. Symptoms may include weakness, confusion, and muscular spasms.

Manganese

- *Good to know:* Deficiency and toxicity are rare in the U.S.

- *Recommendations:* Safe and adequate amounts, ages 11–51+: 2–5 milligrams/day.

- *Benefits:* Part of many body enzymes.

- *Food sources:* Widely available in foods, especially nuts, leafy green vegetables, tea, and unrefined cereals and grain products.

- *Day's supply in:* Any combination of healthy foods.

- *Watch out:* No warnings.

Molybdenum

- *Good to know:* Deficiency and toxicity are rare in the U.S.

- *Recommendations:* Safe and adequate amounts for ages 11–51+: 75–250 micrograms/day.

- *Benefits:* Part of many body enzymes.

- *Food sources:* Milk, legumes, liver, unrefined cereals and grain products.

- *Day's supply in:* Usually attained in the course of a healthy diet.

- *Watch out:* No warnings.

Phosphorus

- *Good to know:* The second most abundant mineral in the body, after calcium.

- *Recommendations:*

    Ages 9–18, 1250 milligrams/day
    Ages 19–70, 700 milligrams/day

- *Benefits:* Works with calcium to form bones and teeth, helps create energy in the body, is part of cell membranes. Phosphorus is present in DNA and RNA, the body's genetic material.

- *Food sources:* Most prevalent in protein-rich foods, such as meat, poultry, fish, eggs, and milk.

- *Day's supply in:* 1 chicken breast (392 mg) PLUS 1 cup skim milk (247 mg) PLUS 1 egg (89 mg).

- *Watch out:* Too much phosphorus can deplete calcium in the blood. Avoid excess consumption of soft drinks, which contain phosphorus.

Potassium

- *Good to know:* People who eat the recommended five servings a day of fruits and vegetables usually get enough potassium in their diets.

- *Recommendations:*

    Adult minimum: 2000 milligrams/day

- *Benefits:* Important for nerve transmission, muscle contraction, and balance of fluids in the body.

- *Food sources:* Many types of fresh foods, including meat, milk, whole grain products, fruits, legumes, potatoes.

- *Day's supply in:* 4 ounce sirloin steak (400 mg) PLUS 1 cup milk (400 mg) PLUS ½ cup kidney beans (329 mg) PLUS 1 baked potato with skin (844 mg) PLUS 1 slice whole wheat bread (70 mg).

- *Watch out:* Excess vomiting or diarrhea, and drugs such as steroids or diuretics may deplete the body of potassium. Potassium supplements are often prescribed along with these medications. Symptoms of potassium deficiency include muscle weakness, confusion, and fatigue.

Selenium

- *Good to know:* Selenium is currently being investigated for its potential to prevent cancer.

- *Recommendations:*
  Ages 15–18, 50 micrograms/day
  Men ages 19–51+, 70 micrograms/day
  Women ages 19–51+, 55 micrograms/day

- *Benefits:* Powerful antioxidant that works to protect cells from damage, important for cell growth.

- *Food sources:* Seafood, meats, grain products, seeds.

- *Day's supply in:* 1 chicken breast (47 mcg) PLUS 1 egg (15 mcg) PLUS 1 slice whole wheat bread (10 mcg).

- *Watch out:* Taking high doses, 1 milligram or higher, can cause toxicity symptoms, including nausea, diarrhea, fatigue, nerve damage, hair loss, and nail changes.

Sodium

- *Good to know:* Sodium supplementation is rarely necessary, even under normal conditions of exercise and sweating.

- *Recommendations:*

    Adult minimum: 500 milligrams/day

- *Benefits:* Important for nerve transmission, muscle contraction, and balance of fluids in the body.

- *Food sources:* Table salt, soy sauce, processed foods.

- *Day's supply in:* The recommended minimum amount is satisfied in daily diet.

- *Watch out:* Too much sodium in the diet has been linked to hypertension in some people who have a genetic sensitivity. Most people get far too much sodium in their diets, due mainly to over-use of table salt. It is recommended that adults aim to keep their total sodium intake below 2400 milligrams per day, or about 1 teaspoon of salt.

Zinc

- *Good to know:* Although some people suggest using zinc supplements to fight the common cold, results of scientific studies have been contradictory.

- *Recommendations:*

    Men ages 11–51+, 15 milligrams/day
    Women ages 11–51+, 12 milligrams/day

- *Benefits:* Part of many enzymes in the body, helps with tissue growth and wound healing, important for taste perception.

- *Food sources:* Protein-rich foods, including meat, poultry, fish.

- *Day's supply in:* 1 small extra-lean hamburger (7.29 mg) PLUS 1 cup chickpeas (2.51 mg) PLUS 1 cup milk (0.98 mg) PLUS 2 slices whole wheat bread (1.1 mg) PLUS 1 cup plain yogurt (2.18 mg) PLUS 2 eggs (1.0 mg).

- *Watch out:* People over age 65 have a greater risk of deficiency due to a reduced ability to absorb zinc, disease states, or use of diuretics or iron supplements. Zinc supplements may be required if symptoms appear, including anorexia, slow wound healing, impaired taste sensation or reduced immune function.

Chapter 3

Calcium: Your Body Needs It

Unearthed skeletons from ancient times testify to the durability of bone long after other bodily tissue turns to dust. Living bone in the body, however, can lose mineral and fracture easily if neglected—a disorder called osteoporosis, or porous bones. One in two women and one in eight men over 50 suffer such fractures, including sometimes life-threatening hip fractures.

But during your preteen and teenage years, you can reduce your risk of fractured bones later in life with calcium-rich foods and physical activity.

Bone Behavior

Your body's 206 living bones continually undergo a buildup, breakdown process called remodeling.

The body starts to form most of its bone mass before puberty, the beginning of sexual development, building 75 to 85 percent of the skeleton during adolescence. Women reach their peak bone mass by around age 25 to 30, while men build bone until about age 30 to 35. The amount of peak bone mass you reach depends largely on your genes. Then gradually, with age, the breakdown outpaces the buildup, and in late middle age bone density lessens when needed calcium is withdrawn from bone for such tasks as blood clotting and muscle contractions, including beating by the heart.

About This Chapter: The text in this chapter is from "Bone Builders: Support Your Bones with Healthy Habits," by Dixie Farley, in *FDA Consumer*, September-October 1997.

"You can't do anything about the genes you're dealt," says Mona Calvo, Ph.D., a calcium expert for the Food and Drug Administration. "As a teenager, though, you can make the most of things you do control that can build your bones and help reduce the risk of fractures when you are older."

Supporting the skeleton with healthful habits now so it can support you later in life is especially important if you

> ✎ **Weird Words**
>
> Calcium: A mineral used for building bones and teeth and in maintaining bone strength. Calcium is also used in muscle contraction, blood clotting, and maintenance of cell membranes.
>
> Osteoporosis: A disease in which bone mass is reduced and the risk of fractures is increased.
>
> Remodeling: The continual buildup-breakdown process by which bones grow and adapt to body changes.

have an increased risk of osteoporosis—for example, if you're female or have a thin, small-boned frame. These habits are proper diet, exercise, and avoiding bone risks—lifestyle choices that are bad for bone, like smoking.

Eat Your Way To Strong Bones

The main mineral in bones is calcium, one of whose functions is to add strength and stiffness to bones, which they need to support the body. To lengthen long bones during growth, the body builds a scaffold of protein and fills this in with calcium-rich mineral. From the time you're 11 until you're 24, you need about 1,200 milligrams (mg) of calcium each day.

Adolescent bodies are tailor-made to "bone up" on calcium. Calvo says that with the start of puberty, "your body is at a higher capacity to absorb and retain calcium."

Bone also needs vitamin D, to move calcium from the intestine to the bloodstream and into bone. You can get vitamin D from short, normal day-to-day exposure of your arms and legs to sun and from foods fortified with the vitamin. Also needed are vitamin A, vitamin C, magnesium, and zinc, as well as protein for the growing bone scaffold.

Mother Nature provides many foods with these nutrients. One stands out, however, as "almost a perfect package," according to Calvo. "Milk is rich in calcium and high-quality protein. Nearly all U.S. milk has vitamins D and A added. And it has magnesium and zinc."

Still, as excellent as milk is for bones, it and other dairy products are not the only foods that contain calcium. All groups in the Food Guide Pyramid, in fact, offer calcium sources—from the pyramid's grain-based foods that you need the most of, to the produce and high-protein groups in the middle, and even to the fats and sweets "use sparingly" group at the top. The importance of choosing calcium sources from the different food groups is that each group offers its unique package of other nutrients as well.

To learn how much calcium is in a food, you can read the food label's Nutrition Facts panel. Look for the "percent Daily Value" (%DV) set by FDA for calcium. The calcium DV is 1,000 mg. But if you are 11 to 24 years old, your growing bones need more—the recommended 1,200 mg. So, each day's calcium %DVs in the foods you eat should add up to 120 percent.

Because many foods are now fortified with calcium, your investigation of labels may turn up surprising sources. To identify foods with at least 10%DV of calcium per serving, FDA allows these terms on their labels:

♣ **It's A Fact!!**

Some things that place you at increased risk of osteoporosis include:

- if you're female

- if you have a thin, small-boned frame

- if you don't eat a proper diet

- if you don't exercise

- if you smoke

- 20%DV or more: "High in Calcium," "Rich in Calcium," "Excellent Source of Calcium"

- 10% to 19%DV: "Contains Calcium," "Provides Calcium," "Good Source of Calcium"

- 10%DV calcium or more added: "Calcium-Enriched," "Calcium-Fortified," "More Calcium."

♣ It's A Fact!!

Girls Need More Calcium

Between the ages 11 and 24, people need at least 1,200 milligrams (mg) of calcium every day. A 1995 survey by the U.S. Department of Agriculture, however, found that girls and young women 12 to 19 got only 777 mg of the mineral daily, overall. Intake by boys and young men in the same age group was 1,176 mg daily.

Daily calcium intake by preteen girls was far short of the recommended level also in 1990-1992 and fell with age, wrote Ann Albertson, M.S., R.D., and others recently in the *Journal of Adolescent Health*. Calcium consumption was only 781 mg at ages 11 to 12, 751 mg at ages 13 to 14, and a mere 602 mg—barely half what it should be—at ages 15 to 18.

Why Is Calcium Intake In Girls And Young Women So Low?

USDA's Agricultural Economic Report No. 746 gives some clues. Compared with other children, female adolescents:

- drink the least amount of fluid milk

- have the highest tendency to skip morning meals, which offer the most calcium because of milk and cereals

- have the highest share of calories from fast-food places, which have a calcium density much lower than foods prepared at home, schools or restaurants.

—by Dixie Farley

An easy daily plan is to drink a calcium source at every meal and eat one calcium food as a snack, says Ruth Welch, a registered dietitian with FDA.

If the lactose sugar in dairy products causes problems like gas, bloating, or diarrhea, try lactose-reduced or lactose-free milk. When fortified, these products can have up to 50%DV for calcium in one serving. Also available are lactase drops and tablets, which can help you digest dairy products like ice milk, yogurt, and cheese.

♣ It's A Fact!!

From the time you're 11 until you're 24, you need about 1,200 milligrams (mg) of calcium each day.

Get Enough Weight-Bearing Exercise

Growing bone is especially sensitive to the impact of weight and pull of muscle during exercise, and responds by building stronger, denser bones. That's why it's especially important when you're growing a lot to be physically active on a regular basis.

And as far as bone is concerned, Calvo says impact activity like jumping up and down appears to be the best. "But the important thing is to get off the couch and get moving at some activity. It really is a matter of 'Use it now, or lose it later'."

Such activities include sports and exercise, including football, basketball, baseball, jogging, dancing, jumping rope, inline skating, skateboarding, bicycling, ballet, hiking, skiing, karate, swimming, rowing a canoe, bowling, and weight-training. And when your parents make you mow the lawn, rake leaves, or wash and wax the car, they're doing your muscles and bones a favor.

FDA's Welch adds, "Day-to-day activities that start in the teen years, like walking the dog or using stairs instead of elevators, can become life-long habits for healthy bones."

✔ **Quick Tip**

Eat Enough Calcium

To get enough calcium for growing bones, each day you need to eat foods whose %Daily Value for calcium adds up to 120 percent. Because the amount of calcium in foods can vary, read the food label check the %DV for calcium in what you eat.

So your body will have all the other nutrients it needs, too, be sure to eat the recommended number of servings from the food groups that make up the Food Guide Pyramid:

- Grain Products Group: 6-11 servings
- Vegetables Group: 3-5 servings
- Fruits Group: 2-4 servings
- Milk Products Group: 2-3 servings
- Meat and Bean Group: 2-3 servings
- Fats, Oils, and Sweets: Use sparingly

As shown below, each group includes foods that provide calcium. The food examples are listed by their serving size and %DV for calcium.

Grain Products

waffles (4-inch square)	2 waffles	20%DV
pancakes (5-inch)	3 pancakes	20%DV
calcium-fortified cereal	1 cup	15%DV
calcium-fortified bread	1 slice	8%DV
corn tortilla	3 tortillas	8%DV
bread	1 slice	4%DV

Vegetables

collards	1/2 cup	20%DV
turnip greens	2/3 cup	15%DV
kale	2/3 cup	10%DV
bok choy	1/2 cup	10%DV
broccoli	1 stalk	6%DV
carrot	1 medium carrot	2%DV

Fruits

calcium-fortified orange juice	1 cup	30%DV
dried figs	2 figs	6%DV
orange	1 orange	4%DV
kiwi	2 kiwis	4%DV
strawberries	8 berries	2%DV

Milk Products

nonfat milk, calcium-fortified	1 cup	40%DV
yogurt	1 cup	35%DV
milk, whole, 2%, 1%, skim	1 cup	30%DV
cheese	1 ounce	20%DV
cheese spread	2 Tbsp.	15%DV
pudding	1/2 cup	10%DV
frozen yogurt	1/2 cup	10%DV
cottage cheese	1/2 cup	6%DV

Meat and Beans

calcium-processed tofu	3 oz.	60%DV
dry-roasted almonds	1/4 cup	10%DV
scrambled eggs	2 eggs	8%DV
baked beans with sauce	1/2 cup	8%DV
black-eyed peas	1/2 cup	2%DV

Fats, Oils, and Sweets

milk chocolate	1.5-ounce bar	8%DV

Mixed Dishes

cheese pizza (12-inch)	1/4 pizza	25%DV
macaroni and cheese	1 cup	25%DV
grilled cheese sandwich	1 sandwich	25%DV
lasagna	1 cup	25%DV
soups prepared with milk	1 cup	15%DV
chili con carne with beans	1 cup	10%DV
taco with cheese	1 taco	10%DV
tuna salad sandwich	1 sandwich	8%DV
chicken noodle soup	1 cup	2%DV

(Source: "Calcium! Do You Get It?" pilot education program funded by FDA's Office of Women's Health)

Avoid Bone Risks

Some habits in the teenage years can steal calcium from your bones or increase the need for it, weakening the skeleton for life.

Skipping meals is risky for bone, Welch says. In our three-meal-a-day society, skipping a meal may reduce by a third your chance of getting your 120%DV for calcium—simply by eliminating one occasion to eat.

Replacing milk with nondairy drinks like soda pop or fruit-flavored teas or drinks is another eating habit that prevents bones from getting the calcium and other nutrients they need.

In a survey comparing 1994 daily beverage intakes with those in the late 1970s, the U.S. Department of Agriculture found a switch from milk to other drinks among young people:

- Milk drinkers among teenagers dropped from three-fourths to little more than half.
- Two to three times more children and teenagers drank non-citrus fruit juices.
- Teenage boys nearly tripled their intake of soft drinks, three-fourths of them drinking about 34 ounces; two-thirds of teenage girls drank 23 ounces.

Alcohol abuse and cigarette smoking can hurt bone. Calvo says, "Alcohol abuse can cause loss of calcium, magnesium, and zinc in the urine. Many who abuse alcohol also have poor diets and malnourished, weaker bones." Cigarette smoke is also toxic to bone and can influence how much exercise you get because it affects your stamina, she says.

Eating disorders can weaken bone. The repeated vomiting in bulimia and extreme dieting in the appetite disorder anorexia can upset the body's balance of calcium and important hormones like bone-protective estrogen, decreasing bone density. And extreme exercising by young women with or without eating disorders can postpone or stop menstruation, when blood levels of estrogen are reduced.

—by Dixie Farley

☞ Remember!!

Small Changes For Big Benefits

As a disorder of aging, osteoporosis may seem far away for worry when you're 15. But, small changes today for better bones tomorrow may be more important than you might guess.

Laura Bacharach, M.D., of Stanford University, wrote in *Nutrition & the M.D.* [in 1996] that adolescents who make "even a 5 percent gain in bone mass can reduce the risk of osteoporosis by 40 percent." And this is in addition to "immediate benefits of feeling stronger and more fit now with these changes!"

Chapter 4

Trace Minerals

What Are Trace Minerals?

- Is extra zinc really necessary when you're under stress?
- Does everyone need iron supplements?
- Will selenium prevent cancer?
- How important is copper?

All these questions are about nutrients belonging to a group known as "trace minerals." They're called trace minerals partly because they are needed by the body in such very small amounts. Compare the small amounts listed in Table 4.1 with the recommended dietary allowance (RDA) for calcium, which is 800 to 1,200 milligrams per day.

Trace minerals known to be needed by humans are listed in the table along with current recommendations for adequate and safe levels of daily intake, and examples of important food sources. If you regularly eat a balanced diet made up of a variety of foods, there normally is no need to take extra amounts or special supplements to supply these nutrients.

Under certain conditions such as pregnancy, abnormally heavy menstrual flow, or recuperation after surgery, your physician or dietitian may make specific

About This Chapter: Text in this chapter is from "Food and Nutrition Facts: Trace Minerals," by Arlette Rasmussen, Ph.D., R.D., Charlotte Ralff, B.S., and Sue Snider, Ph.D., Delaware Cooperative Extension, Document No. FNF-21, March 1997; reprinted with permission.

recommendations to meet special needs. Otherwise, be careful about supplements. As with many other substances, it's easy to go overboard and get too much of a good thing. However, if you do decide to take a supplement containing trace minerals, check the label and don't take more than about 150% of the RDA, since all trace minerals can be harmful when taken in large amounts. Too much of one can also interfere with how well your body uses others. Remember, with trace minerals, a little goes a long way.

Iron

Iron is especially important for the blood formation and function. Therefore, the need for iron increases when blood is lost on a regular basis, or during rapid growth. In both cases, more blood must be formed either to replace losses or to supply the needs of a larger body. Iron intake needs special attention:

- during infancy, not only because of the rapid growth taking place, but also because milk (which contains very little iron) makes up the main part of the diet;
- during the rapid growth of early childhood;
- during a woman's child-bearing years due to monthly blood losses;
- during and until three months after pregnancy.

Even at these times, a varied diet of ordinary foods can supply the body's needs because other factors increase iron absorption. For example, the more iron your body needs, the more iron it absorbs from the food you eat. Also, the form of iron in meat, poultry and fish is absorbed especially well by the body. In addition, when you include some of these sources in your diet, they promote the absorption of iron from other foods such as breads, cereals, eggs, cheese, legumes and nuts. Foods high in Vitamin C can do this, too. Thus, combinations—like orange juice, toast, and cereal for breakfast, a tuna salad sandwich with tomato juice and several strips of green pepper for lunch, and a serving of broccoli to accompany a cheese omelet or rice/lentil casserole dinner entree plus a section of melon or cantaloupe for dessert—will help your body use the iron in your food to fullest advantage.

Table 4.1. Recommended Dietary Allowances for Trace Minerals

Trace Mineral	Recommended Dietary Allowance (RDA)*	Important Dietary Sources**
Iron	10.0–18.0***	Whole grain products; enriched breads and cereals; meat (especially organ meats), poultry, fish; vegetables and legumes
Zinc	15.0	Meats (especially beef and organ meats), poultry, seafood (especially oysters)
Manganese	2.5–5.0	Whole grain products; nuts
Copper	2.0–3.0	Nuts; organ meats; legumes; whole grain products; fruits and vegetables
Fluoride	1.5–4.0	Fluoridated water; seafood; green leafy vegetables
Molybdenum	0.15 - 0.5	Meats; whole grain products; legumes
Iodine	0.15	Iodized salt; seafood; dairy products
Chromium	0.05–0.2	Meats, meat products; cheeses; whole grain products
Selenium	0.02–0.2	Whole grain products; meats, poultry, fish

* For Adults

** Those listed make especially notable contribution, but trace minerals are present in many other foods in small amounts. These can add up and make a significant contribution to the total daily dietary intake.

*** The RDA for men and for women after menopause is the same, 10 mg; for women during child-bearing years the RDA is 18 mg/day.

Doctors often recommend iron supplements for women during pregnancy, or prescribe them if a blood test shows a need for additional iron. But these are special situations involving a specific length of time. If you are taking an iron supplement (or any other supplement, for that matter) be sure to tell your doctor.

Zinc

Zinc plays an important role in body growth, development, and maturation; in tissue repair; and in resistance to disease. Low zinc intake has been linked to reduced growth (in children) and to delayed wound healing and reduced resistance to infection in adults, especially the elderly.

Does this mean that you can encourage growth, speed up tissue repair or increase resistance to disease and other stresses by taking more zinc, even if

♣ It's A Fact!!

Chromium helps the body use carbohydrates efficiently

Copper helps the body use iron effectively, plays a prominent role in cartilage and bone development, enables body cells to use energy.

Fluoride protects against tooth decay.

Iodine is needed to make thyroid hormone.

Iron is important for blood formation and function.

Manganese helps the body use carbohydrates efficiently and aids in the formation of bone and cartilage.

Molybdenum helps the body use other necessary compounds or handle their waste-products.

Selenium helps protect body cell membranes from deterioration.

Zinc plays a role in body growth, development, and maturation; in tissue repair; and in resistance to disease.

you consume enough zinc in your diet? No, it doesn't work that way. Although inadequate zinc intake increases the likelihood that problems will develop, and an adequate intake protects against these problems, extra amounts don't provide added protection. In fact, some research studies indicate that too much zinc can actually hamper the body's fight against disease. Excess zinc can also interfere with copper absorption; the two compete to be absorbed by the body, so too much of one can crowd out the other.

Poor zinc intake may occur among some groups in the U.S. population. For example, individuals on limited budgets and fixed incomes are more likely to have low zinc intakes because several good food sources of zinc, such as beef and seafood, are expensive. But this situation occurs among high-income groups, too. The reason? Poor food choices and diets that are too limited in the amounts and variety of foods eaten.

Food can supply you with zinc safely. Even though zinc may be less available from plant sources such as whole grain products, legumes, and nuts, these foods can still make important contributions to total zinc intake. Supplemental zinc, if used at all, should be taken with caution. Such supplements should not exceed 150 percent of the RDA, and should probably include copper.

Copper

Copper contributes to several important bodily functions. It helps the body use iron effectively in forming blood; it plays a prominent role in cartilage and bone development; and it is one of several nutrients that enable body cells to use the energy present in carbohydrate, protein, and fat.

Severe copper deficiency is very rare. In most cases it is due to a genetic disease. Even mild copper deficiency is uncommon because of the small amounts needed by the body and because copper is present in so many foods. The risk of mild deficiency may increase if the diet is very limited and if zinc supplements are overused.

Copper is still being studied actively by scientists. You may hear reports of breakthroughs in knowledge about copper. Be careful about accepting isolated reports as fact; wait to find out if what you hear or see in the media is reliable information or just somebody's hunch about a chance observation. (This applies to other nutrition information as well.)

Selenium

Selenium is another trace element receiving a great deal of attention in the press. This is because technology has advanced to the point where research on selenium is possible. Before now, it was difficult to measure the small amounts of selenium involved in body functions. For example, selenium intake in the amounts considered normal and healthy for copper (2 mg to 3 mg) would probably cause severe poisoning. On the other hand, in very small amounts, selenium—along with vitamin E—helps protect body cell membranes from deterioration. This means that many different tissues can be affected by too little (or too much) selenium.

Researchers are looking especially hard at whether selenium might protect against cancer, as some studies with animals suggest. But studies which can be applied to humans are very limited and not at all clear-cut. At present it seems safe to say that adequate intake may be beneficial, but that larger amounts are not necessarily protective. Added to the danger of toxicity from large amounts of selenium is the concern that some selenium compounds may be cancer-causing rather than cancer-preventing. Clearly, we need more precise information about human requirements for selenium and about its relationship to cancer. Currently, most health authorities are very cautious about suggesting both satisfactory and safe levels of selenium supplements.

Can you depend on diet to supply the recommended levels of selenium? In this day and age, it is easy to answer yes to that question. The selenium in plant foods depends on the soil in which they grew, and in animal products, on where their food was grown. Some areas of the United States and other countries have high levels of selenium in the soil, and some areas have low levels. Food products available in our supermarkets come from many different growing areas. As a result, variations in the selenium content of foods from different places "average out" in the diet.

There is little cause for concern except for the unusual case of someone who eats exclusively locally grown foods year-round, a highly unlikely situation.

Analyses of diets in different areas of the United States show the typical selenium content is within the recommended range—another good illustration of how important it is to emphasize a wide variety of food choices in your meals.

What About Other Trace Minerals?

Needs for the other five trace elements listed in Table 4.1 are also likely to be met by eating a reasonably varied diet in amounts that meet energy needs. They serve many different functions in the body. Iodine is needed to make thyroid hormone; chromium and manganese help the body use carbohydrate efficiently for energy; manganese helps in the formation of bone and cartilage; fluoride protects against tooth decay; and molybdenum helps the body use other necessary compounds or handle their waste-products.

Some additional trace elements are being studied as possible requirements for humans. New findings about them as well as about those listed above continue to be revealed. Many questions remain to be answered. For more information, or referral to qualified authorities, contact your Cooperative Extension county home economist.

☞ Remember!!

- Diets consisting of a variety of choices from each of the four basic food groups can supply all the minerals you need and in adequate amounts.

- All trace minerals can be harmful in large amounts.

- If someone recommends that you take special supplements, be sure that person is a qualified health professional with training in nutrition.

- For further information and help with such questions, contact your Cooperative Extension county home economist.

Chapter 5

Dietary Supplements

Facts vs. Fads

You've seen the headlines: "Natural herbs melt pounds away—without diet or exercise!" or "Amazing new discovery boosts athletic performance!" The ads usually claim that a doctor has discovered a new dietary supplement, a miracle substance that will make you thinner, stronger, smarter, or better at whatever you do. Best of all, this supplement works without any real effort—all you have to do is send in your money and swallow what they send you.

Having trouble believing these ads? You're right to be skeptical. There's little evidence that dietary supplements have the effects that they claim—and there is evidence that some supplements can cause serious damage to a user's health, especially when that user is a teen.

What Are Dietary Supplements?

Dietary supplements are products that include vitamins, minerals, amino acids, herbs, or botanicals (plants)—or any concentration, extract, or combination of these—as part of their ingredients. You can purchase dietary supplements in pill, gel capsule, liquid, or powder forms.

How safe are these substances? In many cases, no one really knows. The U.S. Food and Drug Administration (FDA), which normally checks out the safety of food and medicines before they come on the market, does not check on the safety of dietary supplements before they're sold. The FDA has to wait until it receives reports of problems caused by supplements before it can investigate and ban a dietary supplement. This means that if you take an untested supplement, you are serving as the manufacturer's unpaid guinea pig, and risking your own health.

Can Supplements Help Me Be A Better Athlete?

Many athletes take dietary supplements to improve their performances, but claims for these improvements are often exaggerated or not based on

---

✎ Weird Words

Amino Acids: Organic compounds; the building blocks of protein.

Anabolic Steroids: Synthetic derivatives of the male hormone testosterone.

Botanicals: Plant products.

Dietary Supplements: Products made of one or more of the essential nutrients, such as vitamins, minerals, and protein, and including (with some exceptions) any product intended for ingestion as a supplement to the diet.

Herbs: Soft-stemmed plants, often aromatic and used for seasoning or in medicine.

Hormone: A substance produced by an organ, gland, or other body part, that regulates certain organs and bodily functions.

Minerals: Nutrients required by the body in small amounts, such as iron, calcium, and potassium.

Protein: An essential nutrient required for growth, cell structure, and tissue repair; a complete protein contains all the essential amino acids; an incomplete protein contains some essential amino acids.

Vitamins: A class of organic compounds required in small quantities for growth, development, and normal metabolic processes.

scientific evidence. Anabolic steroids, man-made hormones similar to the male hormone testosterone, are unsafe and illegal. "In those large quantities, the steroids that would otherwise be a positive in our system can have some major negative side effects, including heart damage, kidney damage, bone problems, and severe acne," says Jessica Donze, a dietitian at the Alfred I. duPont Hospital for Children in Wilmington, Delaware. Studies also show that steroids may be addictive, and that even small doses can interfere with growth in teens.

Another supplement used by some athletes (including home run sluggers Mark McGwire and Sammy Sosa) is creatine. Creatine is produced naturally in the body but some athletes take large, manufactured doses because they believe it helps build muscles quicker. Creatine does not improve a person's athletic potential; it will not help you become a superstar if you are normally a fair-to-average athlete.

Since creatine is unregulated, there is no standard dose; users have no way of knowing what levels, if any, are safe, especially for teens who are still growing.

Although some people take amino acid (the building blocks of protein) powders to increase muscle, "all of those amino acids that they sell at very high cost in a powder you can also break down from the proteins that we eat in our diet," Donze says. "Researchers have shown that simply eating more protein or more amino acids does not lead to increased muscle building. It's exercise that determines your muscle building, not intake."

Some people consider energy bars to be a dietary supplement. Energy bars—a carbohydrate treat often fortified with vitamins—can boost your energy over an extended period. "The advantage of [these] bars is that they're easily preserved and they don't irritate the stomach," Donze says. Just remember to only use energy bars as a snack, not to replace a meal.

Can Supplements Help Me Lose Weight?

If you'd like to lose a few pounds, you might be tempted to try some of the many herbal weight-loss products available today. But none of these herbal remedies work—and some have serious side effects. For example, the herb ephedra (also called Ma huang or herbal fen-phen) is supposed to speed your metabolism. What it really does, however, is cause dizziness, jitters, insomnia (difficulty sleeping), and heart problems. Some users have had strokes, heart attacks, and seizures. Herbs like chickweed, ginseng, kelp, and bee pollen, often included in diet aids, do nothing to promote weight loss—and some can be harmful or deadly in large doses. The only safe and effective way to take off excess pounds remains healthy eating and exercise. If you are concerned about your weight, talk to a doctor or dietitian. He or she can help you get to your healthy weight.

Do I Need To Take Vitamin And Mineral Supplements?

The best way to get your daily dose of vitamins and minerals is by eating a balanced diet that follows the Food Guide Pyramid. But what if your diet consists mainly of pizza and soda? "In general, there's nothing wrong with a teen taking a good solid multivitamin," Donze says. "But it shouldn't be anything really fancy. An ordinary one-a-day vitamin is fine; you don't have to get natural vitamins from a health food store."

Teens should talk to their doctors about additional vitamin and mineral supplements. If you don't like dairy products or if you drink a lot of cola (which can interfere with calcium absorption), you might need a calcium supplement. Vegetarians might want to take vitamin B_{12} (found mainly in food that comes from animals). Teens put on weight-loss diets of less than 1,000 calories a day by their doctors or dietitians, or teens with food allergies, should also discuss vitamin and mineral needs with their doctors.

What about taking large doses of vitamins? This practice can be dangerous. Although water-soluble vitamins (such as vitamin C) will leave your system harmlessly through urine or sweat, the fat-soluble vitamins (vitamins A, D, E, and K) can build up in your body with serious side effects. For example, teens taking oral acne medicines, which contain large dosages of vitamin A, should not take additional vitamin A. Overdoses of vitamin A can cause side effects ranging from headaches and blurred vision to loss of hair and liver damage.

Supplement Warning Signals

Check with your doctor before you take any dietary supplement, including vitamins and minerals. If your doctor starts you on a supplement, watch for warning signals that could indicate problems: stomach or bowel discomfort, pain, headache, rashes, or even vague symptoms like tiredness, dizziness, or lethargy.

And don't believe everything you read or hear. "When it comes to supplements, teens need to be skeptical consumers," Donze says. "The most valuable thing they can do for themselves is to think, 'Oh, really?' and ask questions of people they respect. "Watch out for the Internet—a lot of sites that seem to be legitimate are really trying to sell you something. As Donze explains, "We all love to look for the quick fix. But if it looks too easy, it probably is."

Information From The U.S. Food And Drug Administration

In 1996 alone, consumers spent more than $6.5 billion on dietary supplements, according to Packaged Facts Inc., a market research firm in New York City. But even with all the business they generate, consumers still ask questions about dietary supplements: Can their claims be trusted? Are they safe? Does the Food and Drug Administration (FDA) approve them?

Many of these questions come in the wake of the 1994 Dietary Supplement Health and Education Act, or DSHEA, which set up a new framework for FDA regulation of dietary supplements. It also created an office in the National Institutes of Health to coordinate research on dietary supplements, and it called on President Clinton to set up an independent dietary supplement commission to report on the use of claims in dietary supplement labeling.

In passing DSHEA, Congress recognized first, that many people believe dietary supplements offer health benefits and second, that consumers want a greater opportunity to determine whether supplements may help them. The law essentially gives dietary supplement manufacturers freedom to market more products as dietary supplements and provide information about their products' benefits—for example, in product labeling.

The Council for Responsible Nutrition, an organization of manufacturers of dietary supplements and their suppliers, welcomes the change. "Our philosophy has been ... to maintain consumer access to products and access to information [so that consumers can] make informed choices," says John Cordaro, the group's president and chief executive officer.

But in choosing whether to use dietary supplements, FDA answers consumers' questions by noting that under DSHEA, FDA's requirement for premarket review of dietary supplements is less than that over other products it regulates, such as drugs and many additives used in conventional foods.

This means that consumers and manufacturers have responsibility for checking the safety of dietary supplements and determining the truthfulness of label claims.

What Is A Dietary Supplement?

Traditionally, dietary supplements referred to products made of one or more of the essential nutrients, such as vitamins, minerals, and protein. But DSHEA broadens the definition to include, with some exceptions, any product intended for ingestion as a supplement to the diet. This includes vitamins; minerals; herbs, botanicals, and other plant-derived substances; and amino acids (the individual building blocks of protein) and concentrates, metabolites, constituents and extracts of these substances.

It's easy to spot a supplement because DSHEA requires manufacturers to include the words "dietary supplement" on product labels. Also, [since March 1999, a "Supplement Facts" panel is] required on the labels of most dietary supplements.

Dietary supplements come in many forms, including tablets, capsules, powders, softgels, gelcaps, and liquids. Though commonly associated with health food stores, dietary supplements also are sold in grocery, drug and national discount chain stores, as well as through mail-order catalogs, TV programs, the Internet, and direct sales.

FDA oversees safety, manufacturing and product information, such as claims, in a product's labeling, package inserts, and accompanying literature. The Federal Trade Commission (FTC) regulates the advertising of dietary supplements.

♣ It's A Fact!!

Information on the labels of dietary supplements includes:

- Statement of identity (for example, "ginseng")

- Net quantity of contents (for example, "60 capsules")

- Structure-function claim and the statement "This statement has not been evaluated by the Food and Drug Administration. This product is not intended to diagnose, treat, cure, or prevent any disease."

- Directions for use (for example, "Take one capsule daily.")

- Supplement Facts panel (lists serving size, amount, and active ingredient)

- Other ingredients in descending order of predominance and by common name or proprietary blend.

- Name and place of business of manufacturer, packer or distributor. This is the address to write for more product information.

Dietary supplements are not drugs. A drug, which sometimes can be derived from plants used as traditional medicines, is an article that, among other things, is intended to diagnose, cure, mitigate, treat, or prevent diseases. Before marketing, drugs must undergo clinical studies to determine their effectiveness, safety, possible interactions with other substances, and appropriate dosages, and FDA must review these data and authorize the drugs' use before they are marketed. FDA does not authorize or test dietary supplements.

A product sold as a dietary supplement and touted in its labeling as a new treatment or cure for a specific disease or condition would be considered an unauthorized—and thus illegal—drug. Labeling changes consistent with the provisions in DSHEA would be required to maintain the product's status as a dietary supplement.

Another thing dietary supplements are not are replacements for conventional diets, nutritionists say. Supplements do not provide all the known—and perhaps unknown—nutritional benefits of conventional food.

✔ **Quick Tip**

Before starting a dietary supplement, it's always wise to check with a medical doctor. It is especially important for people who are:

- pregnant or breastfeeding

- chronically ill

- elderly

- under 18

- taking prescription or over-the-counter medicines. Certain supplements can boost blood levels of certain drugs to dangerous levels.

Varro Tyler, Ph.D., Sc.D., distinguished professor emeritus of pharmacognosy at Purdue University, cites as examples garlic and the supplement ginkgo biloba. Both can thin the blood, which can be hazardous, he says, for people taking prescription medicines that also thin the blood.

In addition to medical doctors, other health-care professionals, such as registered pharmacists, registered dietitians and nutritionists, also can be sources of information about dietary supplements.

Monitoring For Safety

As with food, federal law requires manufacturers of dietary supplements to ensure that the products they put on the market are safe. But supplement manufacturers do not have to provide information to FDA to get a product on the market, unlike the food additive process often required of new food ingredients. FDA review and approval of supplement ingredients and products is not required before marketing.

Food additives not generally recognized as safe must undergo FDA's premarket approval process for new food ingredients. This requires manufacturers to conduct safety studies and submit the results to FDA for review before the ingredient can be used in marketed products. Based on its review, FDA either authorizes or rejects the food additive.

In contrast, dietary supplement manufacturers that wish to market a new ingredient (that is, an ingredient not marketed in the United States before 1994) have two options. The first involves submitting to FDA, at least 75 days before the product is expected to go on the market, information that supports their conclusion that a new ingredient can reasonably be expected to be safe. Safe means that the new ingredient does not present a significant or unreasonable risk of illness or injury under conditions of use recommended in the product's labeling.

The information the manufacturer submits becomes publicly available 90 days after FDA receives it.

Another option for manufacturers is to petition FDA, asking the agency to establish the conditions under which the new dietary ingredient would reasonably be expected to be safe. To date, FDA's Center for Food Safety and Applied Nutrition has received no such petitions.

Under DSHEA, once a dietary supplement is marketed, FDA has the responsibility for showing that a dietary supplement is unsafe before it can take action to restrict the product's use. This was the case when, in June 1997, FDA proposed, among other things, to limit the amount of ephedrine alkaloids in dietary supplements (marketed as ephedra, Ma huang, Chinese ephedra, and epitonin, for example) and provide warnings to consumers about hazards associated with use of dietary supplements containing the ingredients. The hazards ranged from nervousness, dizziness, and changes in blood pressure and heart rate to chest pain, heart attack, hepatitis, stroke, seizures, psychosis, and death. The proposal stemmed from FDA's review of adverse event reports it had received, scientific literature, and public comments. FDA has received many comments on the 1997.

Also in 1997, FDA identified contamination of the herbal ingredient plantain with the harmful herb *Digitalis lanata* after receiving a report of a complete heart block in a young woman. FDA traced all use of the contaminated ingredient and asked manufacturers and retailers to withdraw these products from the market.

DSHEA also gives FDA authority to establish good manufacturing practices, or GMPs, for dietary supplements. In a February 1997 advance notice of proposed rulemaking, the agency said it would establish dietary supplement GMPs if, after public comment, it determined that GMPs for conventional food are not adequate to cover dietary supplements, as well. GMPs, the agency said, would ensure that dietary supplements are made under conditions that would result in safe and properly labeled products.

Some supplement makers may already voluntarily follow GMPs devised, for example, by trade groups.

Besides FDA, individual states can take steps to restrict or stop the sale of potentially harmful dietary supplements within their jurisdictions. For example, Florida has already banned all ephedra-containing products, and other states have said they are considering similar action.

Also, the industry strives to regulate itself, the Council for Responsible Nutrition's Cordaro says. He cites the GMPs that his trade group and others developed for their member companies. FDA is reviewing these GMPs as it considers whether to pursue mandatory industry-wide GMPs. Another example of self-regulation, Cordaro says, is the voluntary use of a warning about ephedra products that his organization drafted. He says that about 90 percent of U.S. manufacturers of products containing ephedra alkaloids now use this warning label.

Understanding Claims

Claims that tout a supplement's healthful benefits have always been a controversial feature of dietary supplements. Manufacturers often rely on them to sell their products. But consumers often wonder whether they can trust them.

Under DSHEA and previous food labeling laws, supplement manufacturers are allowed to use, when appropriate, three types of claims: nutrient-content claims, disease claims, and nutrition support claims, which include "structure-function claims."

Nutrient-content claims describe the level of a nutrient in a food or dietary supplement. For example, a supplement containing at least 200 milligrams of calcium per serving could carry the claim "high in calcium." A supplement with at least 12 mg per serving of vitamin C could state on its label, "Excellent source of vitamin C."

Disease claims show a link between a food or substance and a disease or health-related condition. FDA authorizes these claims based on a review of the scientific evidence. Or, after the agency is notified, the claims may be based on an authoritative statement from certain scientific bodies, such as the National Academy of Sciences, that shows or describes a well-established diet-to-health link. As of this writing, certain dietary supplements may be eligible to carry disease claims, such as claims that show a link between:

- the vitamin folic acid and a decreased risk of neural tube defect-affected pregnancy, if the supplement contains sufficient amounts of folic acid

- calcium and a lower risk of osteoporosis, if the supplement contains sufficient amounts of calcium

- psyllium seed husk (as part of a diet low in cholesterol and saturated fat) and coronary heart disease, if the supplement contains sufficient amounts of psyllium seed husk.

Nutrition support claims can describe a link between a nutrient and the deficiency disease that can result if the nutrient is lacking in the diet. For example, the label of a vitamin C supplement could state that vitamin C prevents scurvy. When these types of claims are used, the label must mention the prevalence of the nutrient-deficiency disease in the United States.

These claims also can refer to the supplement's effect on the body's structure or function, including its overall effect on a person's well-being. These are known as structure-function claims.

Examples of structure-function claims are:

- Calcium builds strong bones.
- Antioxidants maintain cell integrity.
- Fiber maintains bowel regularity.

Manufacturers can use structure-function claims without FDA authorization. They base their claims on their review and interpretation of the scientific literature. Like all label claims, structure-function claims must be true and not misleading.

Structure-function claims can be easy to spot because, on the label, they must be accompanied with the disclaimer "This statement has not been evaluated by the Food and Drug Administration. This product is not intended to diagnose, treat, cure, or prevent any disease."

Manufacturers who plan to use a structure-function claim on a particular product must inform FDA of the use of the claim no later than 30 days after the product is first marketed. While the manufacturer must be able to substantiate its claim, it does not have to share the substantiation with FDA or make it publicly available.

If the submitted claims promote the products as drugs instead of supplements, FDA can advise the manufacturer to change or delete the claim.

Because there often is a fine line between disease claims and structure-function claims, FDA proposed regulations that would establish criteria under which a label claim would or would not qualify as a disease claim. Among label factors FDA proposed for consideration are:

- the naming of a specific disease or class of diseases

- the use of scientific or lay terminology to describe the product's effect on one or more signs or symptoms recognized by health-care professionals and consumers as characteristic of a specific disease or a number of different specific diseases

- product name

- statements about product formulation

- citations or references that refer to disease

- use of the words "disease" or "diseased"

- art, such as symbols and pictures

- statements that the product can substitute for an approved therapy (for example, a drug).

FDA's proposal is consistent with the guidance on the distinction between structure-function and disease claims provided in the 1997 report by the President's Commission on Dietary Supplement Labels.

If shoppers find dietary supplements whose labels state or imply that the product can help diagnose, treat, cure, or prevent a disease (for example, "cures cancer" or "treats arthritis"), they should realize that the product is being marketed illegally as a drug and as such has not been evaluated for safety or effectiveness.

FTC regulates claims made in the advertising of dietary supplements, and in recent years, that agency has taken a number of enforcement actions against companies whose advertisements contained false and misleading information. The actions targeted, for example, erroneous claims that chromium picolinate was a treatment for weight loss and high blood cholesterol. An action in 1997 targeted ads for an ephedrine alkaloid supplement because they understated the degree of the product's risk and featured a man falsely described as a doctor.

Fraudulent Products

Consumers need to be on the lookout for fraudulent products. These are products that don't do what they say they can or don't contain what they say they contain. At the very least, they waste consumers' money, and they may cause physical harm.

Fraudulent products often can be identified by the types of claims made in their labeling, advertising and promotional literature. Some possible indicators of fraud, says Stephen Barrett, M.D., a board member of the National Council Against Health Fraud, are:

- Claims that the product is a secret cure and use of such terms as "breakthrough," "magical," "miracle cure," and "new discovery." If the product were a cure for a serious disease, it would be widely reported in the media and used by health-care professionals, he says.

- "Pseudomedical" jargon, such as "detoxify," "purify" and "energize" to describe a product's effects. These claims are vague and hard to measure,

Barrett says. So, they make it easier for success to be claimed "even though nothing has actually been accomplished," he says.

- Claims that the product can cure a wide range of unrelated diseases. No product can do that, he says.

- Claims that a product is backed by scientific studies, but with no list of references or references that are inadequate. For instance, if a list of references is provided, the citations cannot be traced, or if they are traceable, the studies are out-of-date, irrelevant, or poorly designed.

- Claims that the supplement has only benefits—and no side effects. A product "potent enough to help people will be potent enough to cause side effects," Barrett says.

- Accusations that the medical profession, drug companies and the government are suppressing information about a particular treatment. It would be illogical, Barrett says, for large numbers of people to withhold information about potential medical therapies when they or their families and friends might one day benefit from them.

Though often more difficult to do, consumers also can protect themselves from economic fraud, a practice in which the manufacturer substitutes part or all of a product with an inferior, cheaper ingredient and then passes off the fake product as the real thing but at a lower cost. Varro Tyler, Ph.D., Sc.D., a distinguished professor emeritus of pharmacognosy (the study of medicinal products in their crude, or unprepared, form) at Purdue University in West LaFayette, Ind., advises consumers to avoid products sold for considerably less money than competing brands. "If it's too cheap, the product is probably not what it's supposed to be," he says.

Quality Products

Poor manufacturing practices are not unique to dietary supplements, but the growing market for supplements in a less restrictive regulatory environment creates the potential for supplements to be prone to quality-control problems. For example, FDA has identified several problems where some manufacturers were buying herbs, plants and other ingredients without first adequately testing them to determine whether the product they ordered was actually what they received or whether the ingredients were free from contaminants.

To help protect themselves, consumers should:

- Look for ingredients in products with the U.S.P. notation, which indicates the manufacturer followed standards established by the U.S. Pharmacopoeia.

- Realize that the label term "natural" doesn't guarantee that a product is safe. "Think of poisonous mushrooms," says Elizabeth Yetley, Ph.D., director of FDA's Office of Special Nutritionals. "They're natural."

- Consider the name of the manufacturer or distributor. Supplements made by a nationally known food and drug manufacturer, for example, have likely been made under tight controls because these companies already have in place manufacturing standards for their other products.

- Write to the supplement manufacturer for more information. Ask the company about the conditions under which its products were made.

Reading And Reporting

Consumers who use dietary supplements should always read product labels, follow directions, and heed all warnings.

Supplement users who suffer a serious harmful effect or illness that they think is related to supplement use should call a doctor or other health-care provider. He or she in turn can report it to FDA MedWatch by calling 1-800-FDA-1088 or going to www.fda.gov/medwatch/report/hcp.htm on the MedWatch Website. Patients' names are kept confidential.

Consumers also may call the toll-free MedWatch number or go to www.fda.gov/medwatch/report/consumer/consumer.htm on the MedWatch Website to report an adverse reaction. To file a report, consumers will be asked to provide:

- name, address and telephone number of the person who became ill

- name and address of the doctor or hospital providing medical treatment

- description of the problem

- name of the product and store where it was bought.

Consumers also should report the problem to the manufacturer or distributor listed on the product's label and to the store where the product was bought.

> ♣ **It's A Fact!!**
>
> If you suffer a serious harmful effect or illness that you think is related to supplement use should call a doctor or other health-care provider.
>
> You can also report it to FDA MedWatch by calling 1-800-FDA-1088 or going to www.fda.gov/medwatch/report/consumer/consumer.htm on the MedWatch Website.

Today's Dietary Supplements

The report of the President's Commission on Dietary Supplement Labels, released in November 1997, provides a look at the future of dietary supplements. It encourages researchers to find out whether consumers want and can use the information allowed in dietary supplement labeling under DSHEA. It encourages studies to identify more clearly the relationships between dietary supplements and health maintenance and disease prevention. It urges FDA to take enforcement action when questions about a product's safety arise. And it suggests that FDA and the industry work together to develop guidelines on the use of warning statements on dietary supplement labels.

FDA generally concurred with the commission's recommendations in the agency's 1998 proposed rule on dietary supplement claims.

While much remains unknown about many dietary supplements—their health benefits and potential risks, for example—there's one thing consumers can count on: the availability of a wide range of such products. But consumers who decide to take advantage of the expanding market should do so with care, making sure they have the necessary information and consulting with their doctors and other health professionals as needed.

"The majority of supplement manufacturers are responsible and careful," FDA's Yetley says. "But, as with all products on the market, consumers need to be discriminating. FDA and industry have important roles to play, but consumers must take responsibility, too."

Supplement Your Knowledge

Some sources for additional information on dietary supplements are:

American Dietetic Association
216 W. Jackson Blvd.
Chicago, IL 60606-6995
1-800-877-1655 (Consumer Nutrition Hotline)
http://www.eatright.org

Federal Trade Commission
Public Reference Branch
6th and Pennsylvania Ave., N.W.
Room 130
Washington, DC 20580
(202) 326-2222
http://www.ftc.gov

Food and Drug Administration
Office of Consumer Affairs
HFE-88
Rockville, MD 20857
1-800-FDA-4010 (Food Information Line)
(202) 205-4314 in the Washington, D.C., area
FDA Website: www.fda.gov

—by Paula Kurtzweil

Chapter 6

The Importance Of Fiber

Because it causes gas, bloating, and other uncomfortable side effects, fiber may be the Rodney Dangerfield of food constituents. But with more and more research showing that a high-fiber diet may help prevent cancer, heart disease, and other serious ailments, roughage has started to get some respect.

The problem is that most Americans don't get enough fiber to realize its potential benefits. The typical American eats only about 11 grams of fiber a day, according to the American Dietetic Association. Health experts recommend a minimum of 20 to 30 grams of fiber a day for most people.

The Food and Drug Administration has recognized fiber's importance by requiring it to be listed on the Nutrition Facts panel of food labels along with other key nutrients and calories. And, based on scientific evidence, the agency has approved four claims related to fiber intake and lowered risk of heart disease and cancer.

The most recent claim, approved in January 1997, allows food companies to state on product labels that foods with soluble fiber from whole oats may reduce heart disease risk when eaten as part of a diet low in saturated fat and cholesterol. Foods covered include rolled oats, oat bran, and whole-oat flour.

About This Chapter: The text in this chapter is from "Bulking Up Fiber's Healthful Reputation" by Ruth Papazian, Publication No. (FDA) 97-2313, printed July 1997. The article originally appeared in the July-August 1997 *FDA Consumer*.

FDA concluded that the beta-glucan soluble fiber of whole oats is the primary component responsible for lowering total and LDL (low-density lipoprotein), or "bad," blood cholesterol in diets including these foods at appropriate levels. This conclusion is based on a scientific review showing a link between the soluble fiber in whole-oat foods and a reduction in coronary heart disease risk.

The other three claims, allowed since 1993, are:

- Diets low in fat and rich in fiber-containing grain products, fruits, and vegetables may reduce the risk of some types of cancer.

- Diets low in saturated fat and cholesterol and rich in fruits, vegetables, and grain products that contain fiber, particularly soluble fiber, may reduce the risk of coronary heart disease.

- Diets low in fat and rich in fruits and vegetables, which are low-fat foods and may contain fiber or vitamin A (as beta-carotene) and vitamin C, may reduce the risk of some cancers.

Found only in plant foods, such as whole grains, fruits, vegetables, beans, nuts, and seeds, fiber is composed of complex carbohydrates. Some fibers are soluble in water and others are insoluble. Most plant foods contain some of each kind.

✎ Weird Words

Fiber: A substance in foods that come from plants. Fiber helps with digestion by keeping stool soft so that it moves smoothly through the colon.

Flatulence: Excessive gas in the stomach or intestine; may cause bloating.

Insoluble Fiber: Fiber that does not dissolve in water. Insoluble fiber is found in whole-grain products and vegetables.

Methylcellulose: A fiber-supplement, weight-loss product used to create a sense of "fullness"; banned by the FDA in 1991.

Psyllium: A fiber-supplement product made from the seeds of the psyllium plant.

Soluble Fiber: Fiber that dissolves in water. Soluble fiber is found in beans, fruit, and oat products.

Some foods containing high levels of soluble fiber are dried beans, oats, barley, and some fruits, notably apples and citrus, and vegetables, such as potatoes. Foods high in insoluble fiber are wheat bran, whole grains, cereals, seeds, and the skins of many fruits and vegetables.

Fiber's Health Benefits

What can fiber do for you? Numerous epidemiologic (population-based) studies have found that diets low in saturated fat and cholesterol and high in fiber are associated with a reduced risk of certain cancers, diabetes, digestive disorders, and heart disease. However, since high-fiber foods may also contain antioxidant vitamins, phytochemicals, and other substances that may offer protection against these diseases, researchers can't say for certain that fiber alone is responsible for the reduced health risks they observe, notes Joyce Saltsman, a nutritionist with FDA's Office of Food Labeling. "Moreover, no one knows whether one specific type of fiber is more beneficial than another since fiber-rich foods tend to contain various types," she adds.

Recent findings on the health effects of fiber show it may play a role in:

Digestive Disorders

Because insoluble fiber aids digestion and adds bulk to stool, it hastens passage of fecal material through the gut, thus helping to prevent or alleviate constipation. Fiber also may help reduce the risk of diverticulosis, a condition in which small pouches form in the colon wall (usually from the pressure of straining during bowel movements). People who already have diverticulosis often find that increased fiber consumption can alleviate symptoms, which include constipation and/or diarrhea, abdominal pain, flatulence, and mucus or blood in the stool.

Diabetes

As with cholesterol, soluble fiber traps carbohydrates to slow their digestion and absorption. In theory, this may help prevent wide swings in blood sugar level throughout the day. Additionally, a new study from the Harvard School of Public Health, published in the *Journal of the American Medical Association*, suggests that a high-sugar, low-fiber diet more than doubles women's risk of Type II (non-insulin-dependent) diabetes. In the study, cereal fiber was associated with a 28 percent decreased risk, with fiber from fruits and vegetables having no effect. In comparison, cola beverages, white bread, white rice, and french fries increased the risk.

Heart Disease

Clinical studies show that a heart-healthy diet (low in saturated fat and cholesterol, and high in fruits, vegetables and grain products that contain soluble fiber) can lower blood cholesterol. In these studies, cholesterol levels dropped between 0.5 percent and 2 percent for every gram of soluble fiber eaten per day.

As it passes through the gastrointestinal tract, soluble fiber binds to dietary cholesterol, helping the body to eliminate it. This reduces blood cholesterol levels, which, in turn, reduces cholesterol deposits on arterial walls that eventually choke off the vessel. There also is some evidence that soluble fiber can slow the liver's manufacture of cholesterol, as well as alter low-density lipoprotein (LDL) particles to make them larger and less dense. Researchers believe that small, dense LDL particles pose a bigger health threat.

Recent findings from two long-term large-scale studies of men suggest that high fiber intake can significantly lower the risk of heart attack. Men who ate the most fiber-rich foods (35 grams a day, on average) suffered one-third fewer heart attacks than those who had the lowest fiber intake (15 grams a day), according to a Finnish study of 21,903 male smokers aged 50 to 69, published in the December 1996 issue of *Circulation*. Earlier in the year, findings from an ongoing U.S. study of 43,757 male health professionals (some of whom were sedentary, overweight or smokers) suggest that those who ate more than 25 grams of fiber per day had a 36 percent lower risk of developing heart disease than those who consumed less than 15 grams daily. In the Finnish study, each 10 grams of fiber added to the diet decreased the risk of dying from heart disease by 17 percent; in the U.S. study, risk was decreased by 29 percent.

These results indicate that high-fiber diets may help blunt the effects of smoking and other risk factors for heart disease.

Obesity

Because insoluble fiber is indigestible and passes through the body virtually intact, it provides few calories. And since the digestive tract can handle only so much bulk at a time, fiber-rich foods are more filling than other foods—so people tend to eat less. Insoluble fiber also may hamper the absorption of calorie-dense dietary fat. So, reaching for an apple instead of a bag of chips is a smart choice for someone trying to lose weight.

But be leery of using fiber supplements for weight loss. In August 1991, FDA banned methylcellulose, along with 110 other ingredients, in over-the-counter diet aids because there was no evidence these ingredients were safe and effective. The agency also recalled one product that contained guar gum after receiving reports of gastric or esophageal obstructions. The manufacturer had claimed the product promoted a feeling of fullness when it expanded in the stomach.

An Apple A Day And More

Recent research suggests that as much as 35 grams of fiber a day is needed to help reduce the risk of chronic disease, including heart disease. A fiber supplement can help make up the shortfall, but should not be a substitute for fiber-rich foods. "Foods that are high in fiber also contain nutrients that may help reduce the risk of chronic disease," Saltsman notes. In addition, eating a variety of such foods provides several types of fiber, whereas some fiber supplements contain only a single type of fiber, such as methylcellulose or psyllium.

✔ Quick Tip

A word of caution: When increasing the fiber content of your diet, it's best to take it slow. Add just a few grams at a time to allow the intestinal tract to adjust; otherwise, abdominal cramps, gas, bloating, and diarrhea or constipation may result. Other ways to help minimize these effects:

- Drink at least 2 liters (8 cups) of fluid daily.
- Don't cook dried beans in the same water you soaked them in.
- Use enzyme products, such as "Beano" or "Say Yes To Beans," that help digest fiber.

🖘 Remember!!

To fit more fiber into your day:

- Read food labels. The labels of almost all foods will tell you the amount of dietary fiber in each serving, as well as the Percent Daily Value (DV) based on a 2,000-calorie diet. For instance, if a half cup serving of a food provides 10 grams of dietary fiber, one serving provides 40 percent of the recommended DV. The food label can state that a product is "a good source" of fiber if it contributes 10 percent of the DV—2.5 grams of fiber per serving. The package can claim "high in," "rich in" or "excellent source of" fiber if the product provides 20 percent of the DV—5 grams per serving.

- Use the U.S. Department of Agriculture's food pyramid as a guide. If you eat 2 to 4 servings of fruit, 3 to 5 servings of vegetables, and 6 to 11 servings of cereal and grain foods, as recommended by the pyramid, you should have no trouble getting 25 to 30 grams of fiber a day.

- Start the day with a whole-grain cereal that contains at least 5 grams of fiber per serving. Top with wheat germ, raisins, bananas, or berries, all of which are good sources of fiber.

- When appropriate, eat vegetables raw. Cooking vegetables may reduce fiber content by breaking down some fiber into its carbohydrate components. When you do cook vegetables, microwave or steam only until they are al dente—tender, but still firm to the bite.

- Avoid peeling fruits and vegetables; eating the skin and membranes ensures that you get every bit of fiber. But rinse with warm water to remove surface dirt and bacteria before eating. Also, keep in mind that whole fruits and vegetables contain more fiber than juice, which lacks the skin and membranes.

- Eat liberal amounts of foods that contain unprocessed grains in your diet: whole-wheat products such as bulgur, couscous, or kasha and whole-grain breads, cereals and pasta.

- Add beans to soups, stews and salads; a couple of times a week, substitute legume-based dishes (such as lentil soup, bean burritos, or rice and beans) for those made with meat.

- Keep fresh and dried fruit on hand for snacks.

Chapter 7

Questions And Answers About Sodium

Why Should I Be Concerned About Sodium?

The human body needs sodium to maintain normal blood volume and pressure. Sodium also is necessary for the normal functioning of nerves and muscles. But too much of a good thing can be dangerous. Too much sodium can aggravate high blood pressure in some people and increase the risk of high blood pressure among others. Because high blood pressure increases the risk of heart attacks, strokes, and kidney disease, many people are being asked to eat less sodium. Others are trying to do so voluntarily.

How Much Sodium Is Too Much?

The "safe" amount of sodium varies with each individual. According to the National Academy of Sciences, a safe amount of sodium for adults to eat daily is about 1,100 to 3,000 milligrams. This is the amount of sodium found in ½ to 1½ teaspoons of salt.

What Foods Contain Sodium?

Sodium occurs naturally in many foods and is frequently added during processing, cooking or at the table through the use of salt, condiments, or

About This Chapter: The text in this chapter is from "Questions and Answers about Sodium in Your Diet," originally by Carol Hans, Evelyn Jones Beavers, and Diane Nelson, and revised in 1996 by Elisabeth Schafer, © 1996 Iowa Cooperative Extension Service; reprinted with permission.

sauces. Even though sodium is found in many food items, it may not be easily seen or tasted; for example, sodium is an important substance in baking soda and baking powder. That's one of the reasons it is so easy for us to consume much more sodium than we realize.

✎ Weird Words

Sodium: A mineral required by the body to keep body fluids in balance; too much sodium can cause you to retain water. Here are some of the terms related to sodium currently permitted on food labels:

- *Sodium free*: a trivial amount of sodium per serving

- *Low sodium*: less than 140 milligrams per serving

- *Reduced sodium*: 25 percent less sodium than the regular product

- *Light (sodium)*: 50 percent reduction in sodium content compared to regular products

How Can I Decrease My Use Of Salt?

Over the years we've gotten used to the taste of salted foods. We notice the flavor difference when the amount of salt is decreased. Sometimes—because our taste buds become less sensitive as we grow older— food may taste less salty than it really is. It's important to allow for that natural change and to make small changes as we adjust our eating habits. If a doctor or a dietitian has given you a sodium-restricted diet, you should follow their guidelines.

Otherwise, try these suggestions.

1. Add little or no salt to foods. The amount of salt listed in recipes for soups, sauces, casseroles, and baked products may be reduced or, in some cases, omitted with little effect on the flavor. Reduce the amount you use gradually to give yourself time to adjust to a "less salty" taste. Resist the temptation to add salt to foods when eating.

2. Read labels carefully. Some high-sodium foods do not taste salty. For example, ready-to-eat cereals can range from nearly no sodium to as much as 360 milligrams of sodium per 1 ounce serving. Check the ingredient list for "salt," "sodium," or "soda." The Nutrition Facts label

lists the number of milligrams of sodium per serving; compare the stated serving size with the amount you eat.

3. Watch your use of highly processed convenience foods. Look for the types and brands that are lower in sodium, for example the low-sodium versions of snack crackers, canned soups, and processed meats. Use frozen vegetables instead of canned. Substitute freshly prepared foods whenever possible. Always check the Nutrition Facts food label for the amount of sodium in a serving.

4. Save salty foods for a special treat. Catsup, barbecue sauce, mustard, Worcestershire sauce, olives, and pickles are high-sodium foods that have little nutritional value. Use them sparingly.

5. Consider new, low-sodium products. Because so many people are interested in using less sodium, many new products have been developed. Some may meet your needs, while others may be too expensive. Read labels carefully because some "no-salt" products substitute potassium for sodium. Check with your physician before substituting potassium for sodium. If someone else does your shopping, tell them you're trying to cut back on sodium and ask them to look for low-sodium products.

✤ It's A Fact!!

Sodium levels in selected cereals, milligrams of sodium per serving:

- Grapenuts: 190
- Cooked oatmeal: 0
- Cooked wheat cereal: 0
- Instant oatmeal: 300
- Shredded wheat: 0
- Cheerios: 290
- Wheat Chex: 200
- Corn flakes: 290
- Wheaties: 270
- Special K: 230
- Raisin bran: 180

Sodium levels in selected condiments, milligrams of sodium per tablespoon:

- Catsup, regular: 156
- Catsup, low sodium: 3
- Chili sauce, regular: 227
- Chili sauce, low sodium: 11
- Horseradish, prepared: 198
- Mustard, prepared: 195
- Relish, sweet: 124
- Soy sauce: 1,029
- Worcestershire sauce: 207
- Tarter sauce: 182

Sodium levels in selected non-prescription drugs, milligrams of sodium per dose:

- Alka-Seltzer (blue box): 551
- Alka-Seltzer (gold box): 296
- Bromo-Seltzer: 761
- Metamucil Instant Mix: 10
- Rolaids: 53

✔ Quick Tip

These types of foods are now available in low-sodium form, with reduced salt, or with no added salt.

- Canned vegetables, vegetable
  juices, and sauces
- Canned soups
- Dried soup mixes, bouillon
- Condiments
- Snack foods (chips, nuts, pretzels)

- Ready-to eat cereals
- Bread, bakery products
- Butter, margarine
- Cheeses
- Tuna
- Processed meats

☞ Remember!!

The human body needs salt to function. Sodium is the main component of the body's extra-cellular fluids and it helps carry nutrients into the
cells. Sodium also helps regulate other body functions, such as blood pressure and fluid volume, and sodium works on the lining of blood vessels to
keep the pressure balance normal.

The National Academy of Sciences has determined that the recommended safe minimum daily amount is about 500 milligrams of sodium
with an upper limit of 2,400 milligrams, However, the council has said
that lowering sodium intake to 1,800 milligrams would probably be
healthier.

Many Americans are consuming even higher amounts of salt, up to
6,000 milligrams a day. In the end, wise consumers will choose diets of
moderation in all things, including salt.

Excerpted from "The Salt Controversy," by Alexandra Greeley in FDA
Consumer, *November–December 1997.*

Chapter 8

A Guide To Fats

Once upon a time, we didn't know anything about fat except that it made foods tastier. We cooked our food in lard or shortening. We spread butter on our breakfast toast and plopped sour cream on our baked potatoes. Farmers bred their animals to produce milk with high butterfat content and meat "marbled" with fat because that was what most people wanted to eat.

But ever since word got out that diets high in fat are related to heart disease, things have become more complicated. Experts tell us there are several different kinds of fat, some of them worse for us than others. In addition to saturated, monounsaturated and polyunsaturated fats, there are triglycerides, trans fatty acids, and omega 3 and omega 6 fatty acids.

Most people have learned something about cholesterol, and many of us have been to the doctor for a blood test to learn our cholesterol "number." Now, however, it turns out that there's more than one kind of cholesterol, too.

Almost every day there are newspaper reports of new studies or recommendations about what to eat or what not to eat: Lard is bad, olive oil is good, margarine is better for you than butter—then again, maybe it's not.

About This Chapter: The text in this chapter is from "A Consumer's Guide to Fats," by Eleanor Mayfield, an article that originally appeared in the May 1994 *FDA Consumer*. This version is from a reprint of that article, Publication No. (FDA) 99-2286; it contains revisions made in November 1994, January 1996, and January 1999.

Amid the welter of confusing terms and conflicting details, consumers are often baffled about how to improve their diets. Clearly, though, consumers are interested in obtaining this information. In a poll conducted by Nielsen Marketing Research, people were asked to select the food qualities that were "very important" to them, and knowing which foods were low in fat and cholesterol ranked highest.

FDA regulations enable consumers to see clearly on a food product's label how much and what kind of fat the product contains. Understanding the terms used to discuss fat is crucial if you want to make sure your diet is within recommended guidelines.

✎ Weird Words

Cholesterol: A chemical compound manufactured in the body. It is used to build cell membranes and brain and nerve tissues. Cholesterol also helps the body make steroid hormones and bile acids.

Dietary Cholesterol: Cholesterol found in animal products that are part of the human diet. Egg yolks, liver, meat, some shellfish, and whole-milk dairy products are all sources of dietary cholesterol.

Fat: A chemical compound containing one or more fatty acids. Fat is one of the three main constituents of food (the others are protein and carbohydrate). It is also the principal form in which energy is stored in the body.

Fatty Acid: A molecule composed mostly of carbon and hydrogen atoms. Fatty acids are the building blocks of fats.

Hydrogenated Fat: A fat that has been chemically altered by the addition of hydrogen atoms (see trans fatty acid). Vegetable shortening and margarine are hydrogenated fats.

Lipid: A chemical compound characterized by the fact that it is insoluble in water. Both fat and cholesterol are members of the lipid family.

Lipoprotein: A chemical compound made of fat and protein. Lipoproteins that have more fat than protein are called low-density lipoproteins (LDLs). Lipoproteins that have more protein than fat are called high-density lipoproteins (HDLs). Lipoproteins are found in the blood, where their main function is to carry cholesterol.

Fats And Fatty Acids

Fats are a group of chemical compounds that contain fatty acids. Energy is stored in the body mostly in the form of fat. Fat is needed in the diet to supply essential fatty acids, substances essential for growth but not produced by the body itself.

There are three main types of fatty acids: saturated, monounsaturated, and polyunsaturated. All fatty acids are molecules composed mostly of carbon and hydrogen atoms. A saturated fatty acid has the maximum possible number of hydrogen atoms attached to every carbon atom. It is therefore said to be "saturated" with hydrogen atoms.

Monounsaturated Fatty Acid: A fatty acid that is missing one pair of hydrogen atoms in the middle of the molecule. The gap is called an "unsaturation." Monounsaturated fatty acids are found mostly in plant and sea foods. Olive oil and canola oil are high in monounsaturated fatty acids. Monounsaturated fatty acids tend to lower levels of LDL-cholesterol in the blood.

Polyunsaturated Fatty Acid: A fatty acid that is missing more than one pair of hydrogen atoms. Polyunsaturated fatty acids are mostly found in plant and sea foods. Safflower oil and corn oil are high in polyunsaturated fatty acids. Polyunsaturated fatty acids tend to lower levels of both HDL-cholesterol and LDL-cholesterol in the blood.

Saturated Fatty Acid: A fatty acid that has the maximum possible number of hydrogen atoms attached to every carbon atom. It is said to be "saturated" with hydrogen atoms. Saturated fatty acids are mostly found in animal products such as meat and whole milk. Butter and lard are high in saturated fatty acids. Saturated fatty acids tend to raise levels of LDL-cholesterol ("bad" cholesterol) in the blood. Elevated levels of LDL-cholesterol are associated with heart disease.

Trans Fatty Acid: A polyunsaturated fatty acid in which some of the missing hydrogen atoms have been put back in a chemical process called hydrogenation, resulting in "straighter" fatty acids that solidify at higher temperatures. Trans fatty acids are under study to determine their effects on cholesterol.

Some fatty acids are missing one pair of hydrogen atoms in the middle of the molecule. This gap is called an "unsaturation" and the fatty acid is said to be "monounsaturated" because it has one gap. Fatty acids that are missing more than one pair of hydrogen atoms are called "polyunsaturated."

Saturated fatty acids are mostly found in foods of animal origin. Monounsaturated and polyunsaturated fatty acids are mostly found in foods of plant origin and some seafoods. Polyunsaturated fatty acids are of two kinds, omega-3 or omega-6. Scientists tell them apart by where in the molecule the "unsaturations," or missing hydrogen atoms, occur.

Recently a new term has been added to the fat lexicon: trans fatty acids. These are byproducts of partial hydrogenation, a process in which some of the missing hydrogen atoms are put back into polyunsaturated fats. Some of the hydrogenated fatty acids take on a "straighter" structure: these are the trans fatty acids. "Hydrogenated vegetable oils," such as vegetable shortening and margarine, are solid at room temperature because straightening fatty acids allows them to pack more tightly.

✤ It's A Fact!!

A high level of LDL-cholesterol in the body increases the risk of fatty deposits and plaque clogging the arteries, which can produce atherosclerosis—and possibly a heart attack. Avoiding a diet high in saturated fats can help keep LDL levels down.

Cholesterol

Cholesterol is sort of a "cousin" of fat. Both fat and cholesterol belong to a larger family of chemical compounds called lipids. All the cholesterol the body needs is made by the liver. It is used to build cell membranes and brain and nerve tissues. Cholesterol also helps the body produce steroid hormones needed for body regulation, including processing food, and bile acids needed for digestion.

People don't need to consume dietary cholesterol because the body can make enough cholesterol for its needs. But the typical U.S. diet contains substantial amounts of cholesterol, found in foods such as egg yolks, liver, meat, some shellfish, and whole-milk dairy products. Only foods of animal origin contain cholesterol.

Cholesterol is transported in the bloodstream in large molecules of fat and protein called lipoproteins. Cholesterol carried in low-density lipoproteins is called LDL-cholesterol; most cholesterol is of this type. Cholesterol carried in high-density lipoproteins is called HDL-cholesterol.

A person's cholesterol "number" refers to the total amount of cholesterol in the blood. Cholesterol is measured in milligrams per deciliter (mg/dl) of blood. (A deciliter is a tenth of a liter.) Doctors recommend that total blood cholesterol be kept below 200 mg/dl. The average level in adults in this country is 205 to 215 mg/dl. Studies in the United States and other countries have consistently shown that total cholesterol levels above 200 to 220 mg/dl are linked with an increased risk of coronary heart disease.

LDL-cholesterol and HDL-cholesterol act differently in the body. A high level of LDL-cholesterol in the blood increases the risk of fatty deposits forming in the arteries, which in turn increases the risk of a heart attack. Thus, LDL-cholesterol has been dubbed "bad" cholesterol.

On the other hand, an elevated level of HDL-cholesterol seems to have a protective effect against heart disease. For this reason, HDL-cholesterol is often called "good" cholesterol.

In 1992, a panel of medical experts convened by the National Institutes of Health (NIH) recommended that individuals should have their level of HDL-cholesterol checked along with their total cholesterol.

According to the National Heart, Lung, and Blood Institute (NHLBI), a component of NIH, a healthy person who is not at high risk for heart disease and whose total cholesterol level is in the normal range (around 200 mg/dl) should have an HDL-cholesterol level of more than 35 mg/dl. NHLBI also says that an LDL-cholesterol level of less than 130 mg/dl is "desirable" to minimize the risk of heart disease.

Some very recent studies have suggested that LDL-cholesterol is more likely to cause fatty deposits in the arteries if it has been through a chemical change known as oxidation. However, these findings are not accepted by all scientists.

The NIH panel also advised that individuals with high total cholesterol or other risk factors for coronary heart disease should have their triglyceride levels checked along with their HDL-cholesterol levels.

Triglycerides And VLDL

Triglyceride is another form in which fat is transported through the blood to the body tissues. Most of the body's stored fat is in the form of triglycerides. Another lipoprotein—very low-density lipoprotein, or VLDL—has the job of carrying triglycerides in the blood. NHLBI considers a triglyceride level below 200 mg/dl to be normal.

It is not clear whether high levels of triglycerides alone increase an individual's risk of heart disease. However, they may be an important clue that someone is at risk of heart disease for other reasons. Many people who have elevated triglycerides also have high LDL-cholesterol or low HDL-cholesterol. People with diabetes or kidney disease—two conditions that increase the risk of heart disease—are also prone to high triglycerides.

Dietary Fat And Cholesterol Levels

Many people are confused about the effect of dietary fats on cholesterol levels. At first glance, it seems reasonable to think that eating less cholesterol would reduce a person's cholesterol level. In fact, eating less cholesterol has less effect on blood cholesterol levels than eating less saturated fat. However, some studies have found that eating cholesterol increases the risk of heart disease even if it doesn't increase blood cholesterol levels.

Another misconception is that people can improve their cholesterol numbers by eating "good" cholesterol. In food, all cholesterol is the same. In the blood, whether cholesterol is "good" or "bad" depends on the type of lipoprotein that's carrying it.

Polyunsaturated and monounsaturated fats do not promote the formation of artery-clogging fatty deposits the way saturated fats do. Some studies show that eating foods that contain these fats can reduce levels of LDL-cholesterol in the blood. Polyunsaturated fats, such as safflower and corn oil, tend to lower both HDL- and LDL-cholesterol. Edible oils rich in monounsaturated fats, such as olive and canola oil, however, tend to lower LDL-cholesterol without affecting HDL levels.

How Do We Know Fat's A Problem?

In 1908, scientists first observed that rabbits fed a diet of meat, whole milk, and eggs developed fatty deposits on the walls of their arteries that constricted the flow of blood. Narrowing of the arteries by these fatty deposits is called atherosclerosis. It is a slowly progressing disease that can begin early in life but not show symptoms for many years. In 1913, scientists identified the substance responsible for the fatty deposits in the rabbits' arteries as cholesterol.

In 1916, Cornelius de Langen, a Dutch physician working in Java, Indonesia, noticed that native Indonesians had much lower rates of heart disease than Dutch colonists living on the island. He reported this finding to a medical journal, speculating that the Indonesians' healthy hearts were linked with their low levels of blood cholesterol.

✔ **Quick Tip**

Government Advice Dietary guidelines endorsed by the U.S. Department of Health and Human Services advise consumers to:

- Reduce total dietary fat intake to 30 percent or less of total calories.

- Reduce saturated fat intake to less than 10 percent of calories.

- Reduce cholesterol intake to less than 300 milligrams daily.

De Langen also noticed that both blood cholesterol levels and rates of heart disease soared among Indonesians who abandoned their native diet of mostly plant foods and ate a typical Dutch diet containing a lot of meat and dairy products. This was the first recorded suggestion that diet, cholesterol levels, and heart disease were related in humans. But de Langen's observations lay unnoticed in an obscure medical journal for more than 40 years.

♣ It's A Fact!!

People living on the Greek island of Crete have very low rates of heart disease even though their diet is high in fat. Most of their dietary fat comes from olive oil, a monounsaturated fat that tends to lower levels of "bad" LDL-cholesterol and maintain levels of "good" HDL-cholesterol.

The Inuit, or Eskimo, people of Alaska and Greenland also are relatively free of heart disease despite a high-fat, high-cholesterol diet. The staple food in their diet is fish rich in omega-3 polyunsaturated fatty acids.

After World War II, medical researchers in Scandinavia noticed that deaths from heart disease had declined dramatically during the war, when food was rationed and meat, dairy products, and eggs were scarce. At about the same time, other researchers found that people who suffered heart attacks had higher levels of blood cholesterol than people who did not have heart attacks.

Since then, a large body of scientific evidence has been gathered linking high blood cholesterol and a diet high in animal fats with an elevated risk of heart attack. In countries where the average person's blood cholesterol level is less than 180 mg/dl, very few people develop atherosclerosis or have heart attacks. In many countries where a lot of people have blood cholesterol levels above 220 mg/dl, such as the United States, heart disease is the leading cause of death.

High rates of heart disease are commonly found in countries where the diet is heavy with meat and dairy products containing a lot of saturated fats. However, high-fat diets and high rates of heart disease don't inevitably go hand-in-hand.

Some research has shown that omega-3 fatty acids, found in fish such as salmon and mackerel as well as in soybean and canola oil, lower both LDL-cholesterol and triglyceride levels in the blood. Some nutrition experts recommend eating fish once or twice a week to reduce heart disease risk. However, dietary supplements containing concentrated fish oil are not recommended because there is insufficient evidence that they are beneficial and little is known about their long-term effects.

Omega-6 polyunsaturated fatty acids have also been found in some studies to reduce both LDL- and HDL-cholesterol levels in the blood. Linoleic acid, an essential nutrient (one that the body cannot make for itself) and a component of corn, soybean and safflower oil, is an omega-6 fatty acid.

At one time, many nutrition experts recommended increasing consumption of monounsaturated and polyunsaturated fats because of their cholesterol-lowering effects. Now, however, the advice is simply to reduce dietary intake of all types of fat. (Infants and young children, however, should not restrict dietary fat.)

—by Eleanor Mayfield

☞ Remember!!

The "bottom line" is actually quite simple, according to John E. Vanderveen, Ph.D., director of the Office of Plant and Dairy Foods and Beverages in FDA's Center for Food Safety and Applied Nutrition. "What we should be doing is removing as much of the saturated fat from our diet as we can. We need to select foods that are lower in total fat and especially in saturated fat." In a nutshell, that means eating fewer foods of animal origin, such as meat and whole-milk dairy products, and more plant foods such as vegetables and grains.

♣ It's A Fact!!

Snack products containing olestra, a fat-based substitute for conventional fats, now appear on store shelves. FDA approved olestra for use in certain snack foods in January 1996. The agency requires all products containing olestra to be labeled with specific health information.

Procter & Gamble Co. developed olestra, which it is marketing under the trade name Olean.

Because of its unique chemical composition, olestra adds no fat or calories to food. Potato chips, crackers, tortilla chips, or other snacks made with olestra will be lower in fat and calories than snacks made with traditional fats.

Olestra may cause abdominal cramping and loose stools in some individuals, and it inhibits the body's absorption of certain fat-soluble vitamins and nutrients. FDA is requiring Procter & Gamble and other manufacturers who use olestra to label all foods made with olestra and to add the essential vitamins, vitamins A, D, E, and K, to olestra.

The following labeling statement will be on all products made with olestra: "This Product Contains Olestra. Olestra may cause abdominal cramping and loose stools. Olestra inhibits the absorption of some vitamins and other nutrients. Vitamins A, D, E, and K have been added."

Like all food additives, olestra's safety was the primary focus of FDA evaluation. For olestra, the safety evaluation focused not only on its toxicity, but also on the product's effects on the absorption of nutrients and on the gastrointestinal system.

Studies of olestra indicated it may cause intestinal cramps, more frequent bowel movements, and loose stools in some individuals. These gastrointestinal effects do not have medical consequences. The required labeling will give consumers needed information to discontinue the product if appropriate.

Clinical testing also indicated that olestra absorbs fat-soluble vitamins (vitamins A, D, E and K) from foods eaten at the same time as olestra-containing products. Studies also demonstrated that replacing these essential nutrients in olestra-containing snacks compensates for this effect. This information will also be included in the product labeling.

In addition to inhibiting the absorption of essential vitamins, olestra reduces the absorption of carotenoids—nutrients found in carrots, sweet potatoes, green leaf vegetables, and some animal tissue. The company's postmarketing monitoring of olestra consumption levels and additional studies will provide FDA with further information about olestra's effects on the absorption of carotenoids. The role of carotenoids in human health is not fully understood, and FDA is continuing to monitor all available scientific research on it.

In addressing these questions, FDA evaluated more than 150,000 pages of data on olestra, drawn from more than 150 studies. Procter & Gamble submitted these data in its original 1987 food additive petition and in several subsequent amendments.

In addition, FDA sought advice from outside experts through its Food Advisory Committee. A special working group of the committee met in public in November 1995 to review and discuss the safety questions about olestra. The working group evaluated data presented by FDA, the company, and organizations and individuals both opposing and supporting olestra's approval. A clear majority of the working group agreed that all major safety issues had been identified and addressed by the FDA review, and that the data provided reasonable certainty that the proposed use of olestra would be safe. A majority of the full Food Advisory Committee reaffirmed that judgment.

—by Eleanor Mayfield

Chapter 9

Keeping Cholesterol Under Control

Cholesterol Is The Jekyll And Hyde Of The Body

Like the literary split personality, cholesterol has a good side because it is needed for certain important body functions. But for many Americans, cholesterol also has an evil side. When present in excessive amounts, it can injure blood vessels and cause heart attacks and stroke.

The body needs cholesterol for digesting dietary fats, making hormones, building cell walls, and other important processes. The bloodstream carries cholesterol in particles called lipoproteins that are like blood-borne cargo trucks delivering cholesterol to various body tissues to be used, stored or excreted. But too much of this circulating cholesterol can injure arteries, especially the coronary ones that supply the heart. This leads to accumulation of cholesterol-laden "plaque" in vessel linings, a condition called atherosclerosis.

When blood flow to the heart is impeded, the heart muscle becomes starved for oxygen, causing chest pain (angina). If a blood clot completely obstructs a coronary artery affected by atherosclerosis, a heart attack (myocardial infarction) or death can occur.

About This Chapter: The text in this chapter is excerpted from "Keeping Cholesterol Under Control," by John Henkel in the January/February 1999 *FDA Consumer* and "Hearty Habits: Don't Eat Your Heart Out," National Heart, Lung, and Blood Institute, National Institutes of Health, NIH Pub. No. 93-3102, September 1993.

Heart disease is the number one killer of both men and women in this country. More than 90 million American adults, or about 50 percent, have elevated blood cholesterol levels, one of the key risk factors for heart disease, according to the National Heart, Lung, and Blood Institute's National Cholesterol Education Program.

While the institute estimates that heart disease killed nearly half a million in 1996, the most recent year for which figures are available, a study published in the *New England Journal of Medicine* in September 1998 says heart disease deaths have declined steadily over the last 30 years. Indeed, between 1990 and 1994, heart disease deaths decreased by 10.3 percent, the study says. From this and other studies, it appears that this is due largely to improvements in medical care after heart attack, a reduction in the number of repeat heart attacks, and better prevention of heart disease development.

✎ Weird Words

Atherosclerosis: A condition in which blood vessels loose their flexibility; cholesterol and other substances, such as fatty matter, build up inside the vessels.

Risk Factor: A behavior or condition that increases one's chance (or risk) of getting a disease.

Step I Diet: A diet plan for lowering blood cholesterol. The Step I diet includes three components: 1) eat a variety of foods; 2) eat less saturated fat—less than 10 percent of daily calories, less total fat—an average of 30 percent of daily calories, and less dietary cholesterol—less than 300 milligrams); and 3) adjust calories to maintain a healthy weight.

Step II Diet: A diet plan for lowering blood cholesterol that allows less saturated fat and dietary cholesterol than the Step I Diet.

Definitions adapted from "Hearty Habits: Don't Eat Your Heart Out," National Heart, Lung, and Blood Institute, National Institutes of Health, NIH Pub. No. 93-3102, September 1993

A key factor in this drop is that the public, patients and doctors today are better informed about the risks associated with elevated cholesterol and the benefits of lifestyle changes and medical measures aimed at lowering blood cholesterol. "Public health initiatives such as the National Cholesterol Education Program have raised consumer awareness, promoted effective interventions, and have likely contributed to the reduction in heart disease deaths." says David Orloff, M.D., of the Food and Drug Administration's division of metabolic and endocrine drug products.

How To Know When Cholesterol Becomes A Problem

Two types of lipoproteins and their quantity in the blood are main factors in heart disease risk:

- *Low-density lipoprotein (LDL)*—This "bad" cholesterol is the form in which cholesterol is carried into the blood and is the main cause of harmful fatty buildup in arteries. The higher the LDL cholesterol level in the blood, the greater the heart disease risk.

- *High-density lipoprotein (HDL)*—This "good" cholesterol carries blood cholesterol back to the liver, where it can be eliminated. HDL helps prevent a cholesterol buildup in blood vessels. Low HDL levels increase heart disease risk.

One of the primary ways LDL cholesterol levels can become too high in blood is through eating too much of two nutrients: saturated fat, which is found mostly in animal products, and cholesterol, found only in animal products. Saturated fat raises LDL levels more than anything else in the diet.

Several other factors also affect blood cholesterol levels:

- *Heredity*—High cholesterol often runs in families. Even though specific genetic causes have been identified in only a minority of cases, genes still play a role in influencing blood cholesterol levels.

- *Weight*—Excess weight tends to increase blood cholesterol levels. Losing weight may help lower levels.

- *Exercise*—Regular physical activity may not only lower LDL cholesterol, but it may increase levels of desirable HDL.

- *Age and Gender*—Before menopause, women tend to have total cholesterol levels lower than men at the same age. Cholesterol levels naturally rise as men and women age. Menopause is often associated with increases in LDL cholesterol in women.

- *Stress*—Studies have not shown stress to be directly linked to cholesterol levels. But experts say that because people sometimes eat fatty foods to console themselves when under stress, this can cause higher blood cholesterol.

♣ It's A Fact!!

Cholesterol levels for kids are defined differently than the levels for adults.

Total Cholesterol

	Ages 2 - 19*	Ages 20 and up
High	200 mg/dL or greater	240 mg/dL or greater
Borderline	170 mg/dL to 199 mg/dL	200 mg/dL to 239 mg/dL
Acceptable	less than 170 mg/dL	less than 200 mg/dL

LDL-Cholesterol

	Ages 2 - 19*	Ages 20 and up
High	130 mg/dL or greater	100 mg/dL or greater
Borderline	110 mg/dL to 129 mg/dL	130 mg/dL to 150 mg/dL
Acceptable	less than 100 mg/dL	less than 130 mg/dL

*These groups apply to those aged 2 to 19, with a family history of either high blood cholesterol or premature heart disease. (Source: "Hearty Habits: Don't Eat Your Heart Out," National Heart, Lung, and Blood Institute, National Institutes of Health, NIH Pub. No. 93-3102, September 1993.)

Though high total and LDL cholesterol levels, along with low HDL cholesterol, can increase heart disease risk, they are among several other risk factors. These include cigarette smoking, high blood pressure, diabetes, obesity, and physical inactivity. If any of these is present in addition to high blood cholesterol, the risk of heart disease is even greater.

The good news is that all these can be brought under control either by changes in lifestyle—such as diet, losing weight, or an exercise program—or quitting a tobacco habit. Drugs also may be necessary in some people. Sometimes one change can help bring several risk factors under control. For example, weight loss can reduce blood cholesterol levels, help control diabetes, and lower high blood pressure.

But some risk factors cannot be controlled. These include age (45 or older for men and 55 or older for women) and family history of early heart disease (father or brother stricken before age 55; mother or sister stricken before age 65).

What Is High Blood Cholesterol?

Cholesterol levels are determined through chemical analysis of a blood sample taken from a finger prick or from a vein in the arm. Home cholesterol kits, first approved in 1993, test only for total cholesterol levels but are as accurate as tests done in a doctor's office, says Steven Gutman, M.D., director of FDA's division of clinical laboratory devices. "These tests can give a consumer very valuable information when screening for high cholesterol," he says. "But they shouldn't be considered substitutes for a test conducted in a doctor's office." He adds that if test results are elevated, consumers should see a doctor right away for a more refined blood analysis. The National Cholesterol Education Program considers cholesterol testing in a doctor's office to be the preferred way because the patient can get advice immediately about the meaning of the results and what to do.

Besides determining total cholesterol levels, doctors often order a lipoprotein profile that shows the amounts of LDL, HDL, and another type of blood fat called triglycerides. This information gives doctors a better idea of heart disease risk and helps guide any treatment.

✔ Quick Tip

Some teens come from at risk families, in which relatives suffered heart disease at an early age and/or high blood cholesterol Such teens should get their cholesterol checked.

Get your cholesterol tested if:

- One of your parents has high blood cholesterol

- One of your parents or grandparents has had heart problems or a heart attack before age 55.

If you don't know your parents' or grandparents' medical history but you have other risk factors for heart disease, you may need to have your cholesterol checked. Ask your doctor or other health professional.

Treating High Blood Cholesterol

When a patient without heart disease is first diagnosed with elevated blood cholesterol, doctors often prescribe a program of diet, exercise, and weight loss to bring levels down. National Cholesterol Education Program guidelines suggest at least a six-month program of reduced dietary saturated fat and cholesterol, together with physical activity and weight control, as the primary treatment before resorting to drug therapy. Typically, doctors prescribe the Step I/Step II diet to lower dietary fat, especially saturated fat. Many patients respond well to this diet and end up sufficiently reducing blood cholesterol levels. Study data reinforce these benefits. For example, a 1998 Columbia University study examined 103 male and female patients of diverse ages and ethnic backgrounds and found that reducing dietary saturated fat directly affected blood cholesterol. For every 1 percent drop in saturated fat, the study showed a 1 percent lowering of LDL in patients.

But sometimes diet and exercise alone are not enough to reduce cholesterol to goal levels. Perhaps a patient is genetically predisposed to high blood cholesterol. In these cases, doctors often prescribe drugs. The National Cholesterol Education Program estimates that as many as 9 million Americans take some form of cholesterol-lowering drug therapy. The most prominent cholesterol drugs are in the statin family, an array of powerful treatments that includes Mevacor (lovastatin), Lescol (fluvastatin), Pravachol (pravastatin), Zocor (simvastatin), Baycol (cervastatin), and Lipitor (atorvastatin). Many doctors say statin drugs have revolutionized patient care.

"These drugs have had a fantastic impact on cholesterol treatment," says Redonda Miller, M.D., assistant professor of medicine at Johns Hopkins University School of Medicine. "They all lower cholesterol levels, but the side effects are minimal."

Statins work by interfering with the cholesterol-producing mechanisms of the liver and by increasing the capacity of the liver to remove cholesterol from circulating blood. Statins can lower LDL cholesterol by as much as 60 percent, depending on the drug and dosage.

Other Drug Treatments

- *Nicotinic acid (niacin)*—This lowers total and LDL cholesterol and raises HDL cholesterol. It also can lower triglycerides. Because the dose needed for treatment is about 100 times more than the Recommended Daily Allowance for niacin and thus can potentially be toxic, the drug must be taken under a doctor's care.

- *Resins*—Doctors have been prescribing Questran (cholestyramine) and Colestid (colestipol) for about 20 years. These "resins" bind bile acids in the intestine and prevent their recycling through the liver. Because the liver needs cholesterol to make bile, it increases its uptake of cholesterol from the blood.

- *Fibric acid derivatives*—Used mainly to lower triglycerides, Lopid (gemfibrozil) and Tricor (fenofibrate) can also increase HDL levels.

- *Aspirin*—Because studies have shown that aspirin can have a protective effect against heart attacks in patients with clogged blood vessels, doctors often prescribe the drug to patients with heart disease.

Though it is impossible to know yet just how many lives cholesterol-lowering therapies have saved, public health experts say awareness efforts

✔ Quick Tip

One of the main ways blood cholesterol can reach undesirable levels is through a diet high in saturated fat and cholesterol. Fatty cholesterol deposits can collect in blood vessels, raising the risk of heart disease.

Drugs, exercise, and other therapies may be prescribed. But in many cases, cholesterol levels can be lowered by revising dietary habits and limiting the kinds of foods known to boost cholesterol, such as those high in saturated fat. This doesn't mean totally eliminating all your favorite foods, such as desserts, says the National Cholesterol Education Program (NCEP). It means taking a more prudent approach to the kinds and amounts of foods you eat.

When elevated cholesterol is first discovered in a person without heart disease, doctors often start patients on the Step I diet recommended by the American Heart Association and NCEP. On this program, patients should eat: 8 to 10 percent of the day's total calories from saturated fat, 30 percent or less of total calories from fat, less than 300 milligrams of dietary cholesterol a day, and just enough calories to achieve and maintain a healthy weight. A doctor or a registered dietitian can suggest a reasonable calorie level. Food labels also are very helpful in determining how much saturated fat, cholesterol, and calories are in various foods.

If the Step I diet doesn't result in desirable cholesterol levels, doctors may try the Step II diet, which changes the daily saturated fat limits to below 7 percent of daily calories and dietary cholesterol to below 200 milligrams. Step II also is the diet for people with heart disease.

In many patients, blood cholesterol levels should begin to drop a few weeks after starting on a cholesterol-lowering diet. Just how much of a drop depends on factors such as how high the cholesterol level is and how each person's body responds to changes made. With time, cholesterol levels may be reduced 10 to 50 milligrams per deciliter or more, a clinically significant amount.

such as the National Cholesterol Education Program are getting the word out to Americans about heart disease, its prevention and management.

—by John Henkel

☞ Remember!!

What you eat is inseparable from how healthy you are, especially the health of your heart. Eat right and you can lower your high blood cholesterol and thus your risk of developing America's number one killer—Heart disease.

What you eat today can affect your body today, tomorrow, and for decades of tomorrows thereafter. To paraphrase a familiar saying: You become what you've eaten. So eat well.

For more information on lowering blood cholesterol through diet or other means, contact:

National Cholesterol Education Program
NHLBI/OPEC
31 Center Drive, MSC 2480
Room 4A-16
Bethesda, MD 20892-2480
(410) 496-7051
Internet: www.nhlbi.nih.gov

Chapter 10

Special Information For People With Food Allergies And Intolerances

Food allergies or food intolerances affect nearly everyone at some point. People often have an unpleasant reaction to something they ate and wonder if they have a food allergy. One out of three people either say that they have a food allergy or that they modify the family diet because a family member is suspected of having a food allergy. But only about three percent of children have clinically proven allergic reactions to foods. In adults, the prevalence of food allergy drops to about one percent of the total population.

This difference between the clinically proven prevalence of food allergy and the public perception of the problem is in part due to reactions called "food intolerances" rather than food allergies. A food allergy, or hypersensitivity, is an abnormal response to a food that is triggered by the immune system. The immune system is not responsible for the symptoms of a food intolerance, even though these symptoms can resemble those of a food allergy.

It is extremely important for people who have true food allergies to identify them and prevent allergic reactions to food because these reactions can cause devastating illness and, in some cases, be fatal.

About This Chapter: The text in this chapter is from "Food Allergy and Intolerances," a fact sheet produced by the National Institute of Allergy and Infectious Diseases (NIAID) in January 1999.

How Allergic Reactions Work

An allergic reaction involves two features of the human immune response. One is the production of immunoglobulin E (IgE), a type of protein called an antibody that circulates through the blood. The other is the mast cell, a specific cell that occurs in all body tissues but is especially common in areas of the body that are typical sites of allergic reactions, including the nose and throat, lungs, skin, and gastrointestinal tract.

The ability of a given individual to form IgE against something as benign as food is an inherited predisposition. Generally, such people come from families in which allergies are common—not necessarily food allergies but perhaps hay fever, asthma, or hives. Someone with two allergic parents is more likely to develop food allergies than someone with one allergic parent.

Before an allergic reaction can occur, a person who is predisposed to form IgE to foods first has to be exposed to the food. As this food is digested, it triggers certain cells to produce specific IgE in large amounts. The IgE is then released and attaches to the surface of mast cells. The next time the person eats that food, it interacts with specific IgE on the surface of the mast cells and triggers the cells to release chemicals such as histamine. Depending upon the tissue in which they are released, these chemicals will cause a person to have various symptoms of food allergy. If the mast cells release chemicals

---

✎ Weird Words

Allergy: Hypersensitivity or an abnormal response to a substance that is triggered by the immune system.

Immunoglobulin E (IgE): A type of protein called an antibody that circulates through the blood.

Intolerance: Hypersensitivity or an abnormal response to a substance that is not triggered by the immune system.

Mast Cell: A specific cell that occurs in all body tissues but is especially common in areas of the body that are typical sites of allergic reactions, including the nose and throat, lungs, skin, and gastrointestinal tract.

in the ears, nose, and throat, a person may feel an itching in the mouth and may have trouble breathing or swallowing. If the affected mast cells are in the gastrointestinal tract, the person may have abdominal pain or diarrhea. The chemicals released by skin mast cells, in contrast, can prompt hives.

Food allergens (the food fragments responsible for an allergic reaction) are proteins within the food that usually are not broken down by the heat of cooking or by stomach acids or enzymes that digest food. As a result, they survive to cross the gastrointestinal lining, enter the bloodstream, and go to target organs, causing allergic reactions throughout the body.

The complex process of digestion affects the timing and the location of a reaction. If people are allergic to a particular food, for example, they may first experience itching in the mouth as they start to eat the food. After the food is digested in the stomach, abdominal symptoms such as vomiting, diarrhea, or pain may start. When the food allergens enter and travel through the bloodstream, they can cause a drop in blood pressure. As the allergens reach the skin, they can induce hives or eczema, or when they reach the lungs, they may cause asthma. All of this takes place within a few minutes to an hour.

Common Food Allergies

In adults, the most common foods to cause allergic reactions include: shellfish such as shrimp, crayfish, lobster, and crab; peanuts, a legume that is one of the chief foods to cause severe anaphylaxis, a sudden drop in blood pressure that can be fatal if not treated quickly; tree nuts such as walnuts; fish; and eggs.

In children, the pattern is somewhat different. The most common food allergens that cause problems in children are eggs, milk, and peanuts. Adults usually do not lose their allergies, but children can sometimes outgrow them. Children are more likely to outgrow allergies to milk or soy than allergies to peanuts, fish, or shrimp.

The foods that adults or children react to are those foods they eat often. In Japan, for example, rice allergy is more frequent. In Scandinavia, codfish allergy is more common.

Cross Reactivity

If someone has a life-threatening reaction to a certain food, the doctor will counsel the patient to avoid similar foods that might trigger this reaction. For example, if someone has a history of allergy to shrimp, testing will usually show that the person is not only allergic to shrimp but also to crab, lobster, and crayfish as well. This is called cross-reactivity.

Another interesting example of cross-reactivity occurs in people who are highly sensitive to ragweed. During ragweed pollination season, these people sometimes find that when they try to eat melons, particularly cantaloupe, they have itching in their mouth and they simply cannot eat the melon. Similarly, people who have severe birch pollen allergy also may react to the peel of apples. This is called the "oral allergy syndrome."

Differential Diagnoses

A differential diagnosis means distinguishing food allergy from food intolerance or other illnesses. If a patient goes to the doctor's office and says, "I think I have a food allergy," the doctor has to consider the list of other possibilities that may lead to symptoms that could be confused with food allergy.

One possibility is the contamination of foods with microorganisms, such as bacteria, and their products, such as toxins. Contaminated meat sometimes mimics a food reaction when it is really a type of food poisoning.

There are also natural substances, such as histamine, that can occur in foods and stimulate a reaction similar to an allergic reaction. For example, histamine can reach high levels in cheese, some wines, and in certain kinds of fish, particularly tuna and mackerel. In fish, histamine is believed to stem from bacterial contamination, particularly in fish that hasn't been refrigerated properly. If someone eats one of these foods with a high level of histamine, that person may have a reaction that strongly resembles an allergic reaction to food. This reaction is called histamine toxicity.

Another cause of food intolerance that is often confused with a food allergy is lactase deficiency. This most common food intolerance affects at least one out of ten people. Lactase is an enzyme that is in the lining of the gut. This enzyme degrades lactose, which is in milk. If a person does not have enough lactase, the body cannot digest the lactose in most milk products. Instead, the lactose is used by bacteria, gas is formed, and the person experiences bloating, abdominal pain, and sometimes diarrhea. There are a couple of diagnostic tests in which the patient ingests a specific amount of lactose and then the doctor measures the body's response by analyzing a blood sample.

Another type of food intolerance is an adverse reaction to certain products that are added to food to enhance taste, provide color, or protect against the growth of microorganisms. Compounds that are most frequently tied to adverse reactions that can be confused with food allergy are yellow dye number 5, monosodium glutamate, and sulfites. Yellow dye number 5 can cause hives, although rarely. Monosodium glutamate (MSG) is a flavor enhancer, and, when consumed in large amounts, can cause flushing, sensations of warmth, headache, facial pressure, chest pain, or feelings of detachment in some people. These transient reactions occur rapidly after eating large amounts of food to which MSG has been added.

Sulfites can occur naturally in foods or are added to enhance crispness or prevent mold growth. Sulfites in high concentrations sometimes pose problems for people with severe asthma. Sulfites can give off a gas called sulfur dioxide, which the asthmatic inhales while eating the sulfited food. This irritates the lungs and can send an asthmatic into severe bronchospasm, a constriction of the lungs. Such reactions led the U.S. Food and Drug Administration (FDA) to ban sulfites as spray-on preservatives in fresh fruits and vegetables. But they are still used in some foods and are made naturally during the fermentation of wine, for example.

There are several other diseases that share symptoms with food allergies including ulcers and cancers of the gastrointestinal tract. These disorders can be associated with vomiting, diarrhea, or cramping abdominal pain exacerbated by eating.

Gluten intolerance is associated with the disease called gluten-sensitive enteropathy or celiac disease. It is caused by an abnormal immune response to gluten, which is a component of wheat and some other grains.

Some people may have a food intolerance that has a psychological trigger. In selected cases, a careful psychiatric evaluation may identify an unpleasant event in that person's life, often during childhood, tied to eating a particular food. The eating of that food years later, even as an adult, is associated with a rush of unpleasant sensations that can resemble an allergic reaction to food.

Diagnosis

To diagnose food allergy a doctor must first determine if the patient is having an adverse reaction to specific foods. This assessment is made with the help of a detailed patient history, the patient's diet diary, or an elimination diet.

The first of these techniques is the most valuable. The physician sits down with the person suspected of having a food allergy and takes a history to determine if the facts are consistent with a food allergy. The doctor asks such questions as:

- What was the timing of the reaction? Did the reaction come on quickly, usually within an hour after eating the food?

- Was allergy treatment successful? (Antihistamines should relieve hives, for example, if they stem from a food allergy.)

- Is the reaction always associated with a certain food?

- Did anyone else get sick? For example, if the person has eaten fish contaminated with histamine, everyone who ate the fish should be sick. In an allergic reaction, however, only the person allergic to the fish becomes ill.

- How much did the patient eat before experiencing a reaction? The severity of the patient's reaction is sometimes related to the amount of food the patient ate.

- How was the food prepared? Some people will have a violent allergic reaction only to raw or undercooked fish. Complete cooking of the fish destroys those allergens in the fish to which they react. If the fish is cooked thoroughly, they can eat it with no allergic reaction.

- Were other foods ingested at the same time of the allergic reaction? Some foods may delay digestion and thus delay the onset of the allergic reaction.

Sometimes a diagnosis cannot be made solely on the basis of history. In that case, the doctor may ask the patient to go back and keep a record of the contents of each meal and whether he or she had a reaction. This gives more detail from which the doctor and the patient can determine if there is consistency in the reactions.

The next step some doctors use is an elimination diet. Under the doctor's direction, the patient does not eat a food suspected of causing the allergy, like eggs, and substitutes another food, in this case, another source of protein. If the patient removes the food and the symptoms go away, the doctor can almost always make a diagnosis. If the patient then eats the food (under the doctor's direction) and the symptoms come back, then the diagnosis is confirmed. This technique cannot be used, however, if the reactions are severe (in which case the patient should not resume eating the food) or infrequent.

If the patient's history, diet diary, or elimination diet suggests a specific food allergy is likely, the doctor will then use tests that can more objectively measure an allergic response to food. One of these is a scratch skin test, during which a dilute extract of the food is placed on the skin of the forearm or back. This portion of the skin is then scratched with a needle and observed for swelling or redness that would indicate a local allergic reaction. If the scratch test is positive, the patient has IgE on the skin's mast cells that is specific to the food being tested.

Skin tests are rapid, simple, and relatively safe. But a patient can have a positive skin test to a food allergen without experiencing allergic reactions to that food. A doctor diagnoses a food allergy only when a patient has a positive skin test to a specific allergen and the history of these reactions suggests an allergy to the same food.

In some extremely allergic patients who have severe anaphylactic reactions, skin testing cannot be used because it could evoke a dangerous reaction. Skin testing also cannot be done on patients with extensive eczema.

For these patients a doctor may use blood tests such as the RAST and the ELISA. These tests measure the presence of food-specific IgE in the blood of patients. These tests may cost more than skin tests, and results are not available immediately. As with skin testing, positive tests do not necessarily make the diagnosis.

The final method used to objectively diagnose food allergy is double-blind food challenge. This testing has come to be the "gold standard" of allergy testing. Various foods, some of which are suspected of inducing an allergic reaction, are each placed in individual opaque capsules. The patient is asked to swallow a capsule and is then watched to see if a reaction occurs. This process is repeated until all the capsules have been swallowed. In a true double-blind test, the doctor is also "blinded" (the capsules having been made up by some other medical person) so that neither the patient nor the doctor knows which capsule contains the allergen.

The advantage of such a challenge is that if the patient has a reaction only to suspected foods and not to other foods tested, it confirms the diagnosis. Someone with a history of severe reactions, however, cannot be tested this way. In addition, this testing is expensive because it takes a lot of time to perform and multiple food allergies are difficult to evaluate with this procedure.

Consequently, double-blind food challenges are done infrequently. This type of testing is most commonly used when the doctor believes that the reaction a person is describing is not due to a specific food and the doctor wishes to obtain evidence to support this judgment so that additional efforts may be directed at finding the real cause of the reaction.

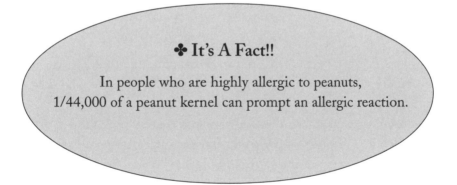

♣ It's A Fact!!

In people who are highly allergic to peanuts,
1/44,000 of a peanut kernel can prompt an allergic reaction.

Exercise-Induced Food Allergy

At least one situation may require more than the simple ingestion of a food allergen to provoke a reaction: exercise-induced food allergy. People who experience this reaction eat a specific food before exercising. As they exercise and their body temperature goes up, they begin to itch, get light-headed, and soon have allergic reactions such as hives or even anaphylaxis. The cure for exercised-induced food allergy is simple—not eating for a couple of hours before exercising.

Treatment

Food allergy is treated by dietary avoidance. Once a patient and the patient's doctor have identified the food to which the patient is sensitive, the food must be removed from the patient's diet. To do this, patients must read lengthy, detailed ingredient lists on each food they are considering eating. Many allergy-producing foods such as peanuts, eggs, and milk, appear in foods one normally would not associate them with. Peanuts, for example, are often used as a protein source and eggs are used in some salad dressings. The FDA requires ingredients in a food to appear on its label. People can avoid most of the things to which they are sensitive if they read food labels carefully and avoid restaurant-prepared foods that might have ingredients to which they are allergic.

In highly allergic people even minuscule amounts of a food allergen (for example, 1/44,000 of a peanut kernel) can prompt an allergic reaction. Other less sensitive people may be able to tolerate small amounts of a food to which they are allergic.

Patients with severe food allergies must be prepared to treat an inadvertent exposure. Even people who know a lot about what they are sensitive to occasionally make a mistake. To protect themselves, people who have had anaphylactic reactions to a food should wear medical alert bracelets or necklaces stating that they have a food allergy and that they are subject to severe reactions. Such people should always carry a syringe of adrenaline (epinephrine), obtained by prescription from their doctors, and be prepared to self-administer it if they think they are getting a food allergic reaction. They should then immediately seek medical help by either calling the rescue squad or by having themselves transported to an emergency room. Anaphylactic allergic reactions can be fatal even when they start off with mild symptoms such as a tingling in the mouth and throat or gastrointestinal discomfort.

Special precautions are warranted with children. Parents and caregivers must know how to protect children from foods to which the children are allergic and how to manage the children if they consume a food to which they are allergic, including the administration of epinephrine. Schools must have plans in place to address any emergency.

There are several medications that a patient can take to relieve food allergy symptoms that are not part of an anaphylactic reaction. These include antihistamines to relieve gastrointestinal symptoms, hives, or sneezing and a runny nose. Bronchodilators can relieve asthma symptoms. These medications are taken after people have inadvertently ingested a food to which they are allergic but are not effective in preventing an allergic reaction when taken prior to eating the food. No medication in any form can be taken before eating a certain food that will reliably prevent an allergic reaction to that food.

There are a few non-approved treatments for food allergies. One involves injections containing small quantities of the food extracts to which the patient is allergic. These shots are given on a regular basis for a long period of time with the aim of "desensitizing" the patient to the food allergen. Researchers have not yet proven that allergy shots relieve food allergies.

Infants And Children

Milk and soy allergies are particularly common in infants and young children. These allergies sometimes do not involve hives and asthma, but rather lead to colic, and perhaps blood in the stool or poor growth. Infants and children are thought to be particularly susceptible to this allergic syndrome because of the immaturity of their immune and digestive systems. Milk or soy allergies in infants can develop within days to months of birth. Sometimes there is a family history of allergies or feeding problems. The clinical picture is one of a very unhappy colicky child who may not sleep well at night. The doctor diagnoses food allergy partly by changing the child's diet. Rarely, food challenge is used.

If the baby is on cow's milk, the doctor may suggest a change to soy formula or exclusive breast milk, if possible. If soy formula causes an allergic reaction, the baby may be placed on an elemental formula. These formulas are processed proteins (basically sugars and amino acids). There are few if any allergens within these materials. The doctor will sometimes prescribe corticosteroids to treat infants with severe food allergies. Fortunately, time usually heals this particular gastrointestinal disease. It tends to resolve within the first few years of life.

Exclusive breast feeding (excluding all other foods) of infants for the first 6 to 12 months of life is often suggested to avoid milk or soy allergies from developing within that time frame. Such breast feeding often allows parents to avoid infant-feeding problems, especially if the parents are allergic (and the infant therefore is likely to be allergic). There are some children who are so sensitive to a certain food, however, that if the food is eaten by the mother, sufficient quantities enter the breast milk to cause a food reaction in the child. Mothers sometimes must themselves avoid eating those foods to which the baby is allergic.

There is no conclusive evidence that breast feeding prevents the development of allergies later in life. It does, however, delay the onset of food allergies by delaying the infant's exposure to those foods that can prompt allergies, and it may avoid altogether those feeding problems seen in infants. By delaying the introduction of solid foods until the infant is 6 months old or older, parents can also prolong the child's allergy-free period.

Controversial Issues

There are several disorders thought by some to be caused by food allergies, but the evidence is currently insufficient or contrary to such claims. It is controversial, for example, whether migraine headaches can be caused by food allergies. There are studies showing that people who are prone to migraines can have their headaches brought on by histamines and other substances in foods. The more difficult issue is whether food allergies actually cause migraines in such people. There is virtually no evidence that most rheumatoid arthritis or osteoarthritis can be made worse by foods, despite claims to the contrary. There is also no evidence that food allergies can cause a disorder called the allergic tension fatigue syndrome, in which people are tired, nervous, and may have problems concentrating, or have headaches.

Cerebral allergy is a term that has been applied to people who have trouble concentrating and have headaches as well as other complaints. This is sometimes attributed to mast cells degranulating in the brain but no other place in the body. There is no evidence that such a scenario can happen, and most doctors do not currently recognize cerebral allergy as a disorder.

Another controversial topic is environmental illness. In a seemingly pristine environment, some people have many non-specific complaints such as problems concentrating or depression. Sometimes this is attributed to small amounts of allergens or toxins in the environment. There is no evidence that such problems are due to food allergies.

Some people believe hyperactivity in children is caused by food allergies. But researchers have found that this behavioral disorder in children is only occasionally associated with food additives, and then only when such additives are consumed in large amounts. There is no evidence that a true food allergy can affect a child's activity except for the proviso that if a child itches and sneezes and wheezes a lot, the child may be miserable and therefore more difficult to guide. Also, children who are on anti-allergy medicines that can cause drowsiness may get sleepy in school or at home.

Controversial Diagnostic Techniques

One controversial diagnostic technique is cytotoxicity testing, in which a food allergen is added to a patient's blood sample. A technician then examines the sample under the microscope to see if white cells in the blood "die." Scientists have evaluated this technique in several studies and have not been found it to effectively diagnose food allergy.

Another controversial approach is called sublingual or, if it is injected under the skin, subcutaneous provocative challenge. In this procedure, dilute food allergen is administered under the tongue of the person who may feel that his or her arthritis, for instance, is due to foods. The technician then asks the patient if the food allergen has aggravated the arthritis symptoms. In clinical studies, researchers have not shown that this procedure can effectively diagnose food allergies.

An immune complex assay is sometimes done on patients suspected of having food allergies to see if there are complexes of certain antibodies bound to the food allergen in the bloodstream. It is said that these immune complexes correlate with food allergies. But the formation of such immune complexes is a normal offshoot of food digestion, and everyone, if tested with a sensitive enough measurement, has them. To date, no one has conclusively shown that this test correlates with allergies to foods.

Another test is the IgG subclass assay, which looks specifically for certain kinds of IgG antibody. Again, there is no evidence that this diagnoses food allergy.

Controversial Treatments

Controversial treatments include putting a dilute solution of a particular food under the tongue about a half hour before the patient eats that food. This is an attempt to "neutralize" the subsequent exposure to the food that the patient believes is harmful. As the results of a carefully conducted clinical study show, this procedure is not effective in preventing an allergic reaction.

☞ Remember!!

Food allergies are caused by immunologic reactions to foods. There actually are several discrete diseases under this category, and a number of foods that can cause these problems.

After one suspects a food allergy, a medical evaluation is the key to proper management. Treatment is basically avoiding the food(s) after it is identified. People with food allergies should become knowledgeable about allergies and how they are treated, and should work with their physicians.

The following organizations can provide more information about food allergies and intolerances:

Hotline:

National Jewish Medical and
Research Center in Denver.
Nurses available to answer
questions
1-800-222-LUNG
http://www.njc.org

Allergy Referrals:

American Academy of Allergy,
Asthma and Immunology
611 East Wells Street
Milwaukee, WI 53202
(414) 272-6071
1-800-822-2762
http://www.aaaai.org

Extracts For Allergy Testing:

U.S. Food and Drug Administration
Center for Biologics Evaluation
and Research
1401 Rockville Pike, Suite 200N
Rockville, MD 20852-1448
1-800-835-4709
http://www.fda.gov/cber

Eczema:

American Academy of
Dermatology
930 N. Meacham Rd.
Schaumburg, IL 60173
(847) 330-0230
1-888-462-DERM
http://www.aad.org/

Eczema Association
1220 S.W. Morrison, Suite 433
Portland, OR 97205
(503) 228-4430
1-800-818-7546
http://www.eczema-assn.org

National Arthritis, Musculo-
skeletal and Skin Diseases
Information Clearinghouse
One AMS Circle
Bethesda, MD 20892-3675
(301) 495-4484
http://www.nih.gov/niams

Lactose Intolerance And Celiac
Sprue:

National Digestive Diseases
Information Clearinghouse
2 Information Way
Bethesda, MD 20892
(301) 654-3810
http://www.niddk.nih.gov/health/
digest/pubs/lactose/lactose.htm
http://www.niddk.nih.gov/health/
digest/pubs/celiac/index.htm

Food Contents:

U.S. Department of Agriculture
Food and Nutrition Information
Center
National Agricultural Library
Agricultural Research Service
10301 Baltimore Ave., Room 304
Beltsville, MD 20705-2351
(301) 436-7725
http://www.nal.usda.gov/fnic

Recipes:

American Dietetic Association
216 W. Jackson Boulevard
Chicago, IL 60606-6995
1-800-877-1655
http://www.eatright.org

Resources:

American College of Allergy,   Food Allergy Network
Asthma and Immunology   10400 Eaton Place, Suite 107
85 W. Algonquin Road, Suite 550   Fairfax, VA 22030-2008
Arlington Heights, IL 60005   1-800-929-4040
1-800-842-7777   http://www.foodallergy.org
http://allergy.mcg.edu

Asthma and Allergy Foundation of
America
1233 20th Street, N.W., Suite 402
Washington, DC 20036
1-800-7-ASTHMA
http://www.aafa.org

Part 2

Dietary Choices

Chapter 11

Dietary Guidelines And Healthy Choices

Eating is one of life's greatest pleasures. Since there are many foods and many ways to build a healthy diet and lifestyle, there is lots of room for choice.

Ten guidelines point the way to good health. These guidelines are intended for healthy children (ages 2 years and older) and adults of any age.

1. Aim For A Healthy Weight

Choose a lifestyle that combines sensible eating with regular physical activity. Being overweight or obese increases your risk for high blood pressure, high blood cholesterol, heart disease, stroke, diabetes, certain types of cancer, arthritis, and breathing problems. A healthy weight is key to a long, healthy life.

Manage Your Weight

Our genes affect our tendency to gain weight. A tendency to gain weight is increased when food is plentiful and when we use equipment and vehicles to save time and energy. However, it is possible to manage your weight through balancing the calories you eat with your physical activity choices.

About This Chapter: The text in this chapter is excerpted from *Nutrition and Your Health: Dietary Guidelines for Americans, Fifth Edition*, 2000, Home and Garden Bulletin No. 232, United States Department of Agriculture (USDA).

To make it easier to manage your weight, make long-term changes in your eating behavior and physical activity. To do this, build a healthy base and make sensible choices. Choose a healthful assortment of foods that includes vegetables, fruits, grains (especially whole grains), skim milk, and fish, lean meat, poultry, or beans. Choose foods that are low in fat and added sugars most of the time. Whatever the food, eat a sensible portion size.

Try to be more active throughout the day. Over time, even a small decrease in calories eaten and a small increase in physical activity can keep you from gaining weight or help you lose weight.

♣ It's A Fact!!

The carbohydrates, fats, and proteins in food supply energy, which is measured in calories. High-fat foods contain more calories than the same amount of other foods, so they can make it difficult for you to avoid excess calories. However, *low fat* doesn't always mean low calorie. Sometimes extra sugars are added to low-fat muffins or desserts, for example, and they may be just as high in calories.

Your pattern of eating may be important. Snacks and meals eaten away from home provide a large part of daily calories for many people. Choose them wisely. Try fruits, vegetables, whole grain foods, or a cup of low-fat milk or yogurt for a snack. When eating out, choose small portions of foods. If you choose fish, poultry, or lean meat, ask that it be grilled rather than fried.

Encourage Healthy Weight In Children

Children need enough food for proper growth, but too many calories and too little physical activity lead to overweight. The number of overweight U.S. children has risen dramatically in recent years. Encourage healthy weight by offering children grain products; vegetables and fruits; low-fat dairy products; and beans, lean meat, poultry, fish, or nuts. Offer only small amounts of food high in fat or added sugars. Encourage children to take part in vigorous activities. Limit the time they spend in sedentary activities like watching television or playing computer or video games.

Help children to develop healthy eating habits. Make small changes. For example, serve low-fat milk rather than whole milk and offer one cookie instead of two. Since children still need to grow, weight loss is not recommended unless guided by a health care provider.

> ✔ **Quick Tip**
>
> If you need to lose weight, do so gradually. If you are overweight, losing 5 to 15 percent of your body weight may improve your health, ability to function, and quality of life. Aim to lose about 10 percent of your weight over about 6 months. This would be 20 pounds of weight loss for someone who weighs 200 pounds. Loss of 1/2 to 2 pounds per week is usually safe. Even if you have regained weight in the past, it's worthwhile to try again.

Serious Eating Disorders

Frequent binge eating, with or without periods of food restriction, may be a sign of a serious eating disorder. Other signs of eating disorders include preoccupation with body weight or food (or both—regardless of body weight), dramatic weight loss, excessive exercise, self-induced vomiting, and the abuse of laxatives. Seek help from a health care provider if any of these apply to you, a family member, or a friend.

2. Be Physically Active Each Day

Being physically active and maintaining a healthy weight are both needed for good health, but they benefit health in different ways. Children, teens, adults, and the elderly—all can improve their health and well-being and have fun by including moderate amounts of physical activity in their daily lives. Physical activity involves moving the body. A moderate physical activity is any activity that requires about as much energy as walking 2 miles in 30 minutes.

Aim to accumulate at least 30 minutes (adults) or 60 minutes (children) of moderate physical activity most days of the week, preferably daily. If you already get 30 minutes of physical activity daily, you can gain even more health benefits by increasing the amount of time that you are physically active or by taking part in more vigorous activities. No matter what activity you choose, you can do it all at once, or spread it out over two or three times during the day.

Make Physical Activity A Regular Part Of Your Routine

Choose activities that you enjoy and that you can do regularly. Some people prefer activities that fit into their daily routine, like gardening or taking extra trips up and down stairs. Others prefer a regular exercise program, such as a physical activity program. Some do both. The important thing is to be physically active every day.

♣ **It's A Fact!!**

Health benefits of regular physical activity:

- Increases physical fitness

- Helps build and maintain healthy bones, muscles, and joints

- Builds endurance and muscular strength

- Helps manage weight

- Lowers risk factors for cardiovascular disease, colon cancer, and type 2 diabetes

- Helps control blood pressure

- Promotes psychological well-being and self-esteem

- Reduces feelings of depression and anxiety

Health Benefits Of Physical Activity

Compared with being very sedentary, being physically active for at least 30 minutes on most days of the week reduces the risk of developing or dying of heart disease. It has other health benefits as well. No one is too young or too old to enjoy the benefits of regular physical activity.

Two types of physical activity are especially beneficial:

- *Aerobic activities.* These are activities that speed your heart rate and breathing. They help cardiovascular fitness.
- *Activities for strength and flexibility.* Developing strength may help build and maintain your bones. Carrying groceries and lifting weights are two strength-building activities. Gentle stretching, dancing, or yoga can increase flexibility.

Physical Activity And Nutrition

Physical activity and nutrition work together for better health. For example, physical activity increases the amount of calories you use. Increasing the calories you use allows you to eat more, which makes it easier to get the nutrients you need. Physical activity and nutrition work together for bone health, too. Calcium and other nutrients are needed to build and maintain strong bones, but physical activity is needed as well.

Children Need To Be Physically Active

Children and adolescents benefit from physical activity in many ways. They need at least 60 minutes of physical activity daily.

3. Let The Pyramid Guide Your Food Choices

Different foods contain different nutrients and other healthful substances. No single food can supply all the nutrients in the amounts you need. For example, oranges provide vitamin C and folate but no vitamin B_{12}; cheese provides calcium and vitamin B_{12} but no vitamin C. To make sure you get all the nutrients and other substances you need for health, build a healthy base by using the Food Guide Pyramid as a starting point. Choose the recommended number of daily servings from each of the five major food groups. If you avoid all foods from any of the five food groups, seek guidance to help ensure that you get all the nutrients you need. [See Chapter 12 for more information on how to use the Food Pyramid.]

Use Plant Foods As The Foundation Of Your Meals

There are many ways to create a healthy eating pattern, but they all start with the three food groups at the base of the Pyramid: grains, fruits, and vegetables. Eating a variety of grains (especially whole grain foods), fruits, and vegetables is the basis of healthy eating. Enjoy meals that have rice, pasta, tortillas, or whole grain bread at the center of the plate, accompanied by plenty of fruits and vegetables and a moderate amount of low-fat foods from the milk group and the meat and beans group. Go easy on foods high in fat or sugars.

> ### ✔ Quick Tip
>
> Choose a variety of foods for good nutrition. Since foods within most food groups differ in their content of nutrients and other beneficial substances, choosing a variety helps you get all the nutrients and fiber you need. It can also help keep your meals interesting from day to day.

There Are Many Healthful Eating Patterns

Different people like different foods and like to prepare the same foods in different ways. Culture, family background, religion, moral beliefs, the cost and availability of food, life experiences, food intolerances, and allergies affect people's food choices. Use the Food Guide Pyramid as a starting point to shape your eating pattern. It provides a good guide to make sure you get enough nutrients. Make choices from each major group in the Food Guide Pyramid, and combine them however you like. For example, those who like Mexican cuisine might choose tortillas from the grains group and beans from the meat and beans group, while those who eat Asian food might choose rice from the grains group and tofu from the meat and beans group.

If you usually avoid all foods from one or two of the food groups, be sure to get enough nutrients from other food groups. For example, if you choose not to eat milk products because of intolerance to lactose or for other reasons, choose other foods that are good sources of calcium, and be sure to get enough vitamin D. Meat, fish, and poultry are major contributors of iron, zinc, and B vitamins in most American diets. If you choose to avoid all or most animal products, be sure to get enough iron, vitamin B_{12}, calcium, and zinc from other sources. Vegetarian diets can be consistent with the *Dietary Guidelines for Americans,* and meet Recommended Dietary Allowances for nutrients.

♣ It's A Fact!!

Growing children, teenagers, women, and older adults have higher needs for some nutrients.

Adolescents and adults over age 50 have an especially high need for calcium, but most people need to eat plenty of good sources of calcium for healthy bones throughout life. When selecting dairy products to get enough calcium, choose those that are low in fat or fat free to avoid getting too much saturated fat. Young children, teenage girls, and women of childbearing age need enough good sources of iron, such as lean meats and cereals with added nutrients, to keep up their iron stores. Women who could become pregnant need extra folic acid, and older adults need extra vitamin D.

Check The Food Label

Food labels have several parts, including the front panel, Nutrition Facts, and ingredient list. The front panel often tells you if nutrients have been added—for example, "iodized salt" lets you know that iodine has been added, and "enriched pasta" (or "enriched" grain of any type) means that thiamin, riboflavin, niacin, iron, and folic acid have been added.

The ingredient list tells you what's in the food, including any nutrients, fats, or sugars that have been added. The ingredients are listed in descending order by weight.

Use the Nutrition Facts to see if a food is a good source of a nutrient or to compare similar foods—for example, to find which brand of frozen dinner is lower in saturated fat, or which kind of breakfast cereal contains more folic

HOW TO READ A NUTRITION FACTS LABEL

Macaroni & Cheese

Nutrition Facts

Serving Size 1 cup (228g)
Servings Per Container 2

Start Here ➡

Amount Per Serving

Calories 250	Calories from Fat 110

% Daily Value*

Total Fat 12g	**18**%
Saturated Fat 3g	**15**%
Cholesterol 30mg	**10**%
Sodium 470mg	**20**%
Total Carbohydrate 31g	**10**%
Dietary Fiber 0g	**0**%
Sugars 5g	
Protein 5g	

Limit these Nutrients

Vitamin A	4%
Vitamin C	2%
Calcium	20%
Iron	4%

Get Enough of these Nutrients

* Percent Daily Values are based on a 2,000 calorie diet.
Your Daily Values may be higher or lower depending on
your calorie needs:

	Calories:	2,000	2,500
Total Fat	Less than	65g	80g
Sat Fat	Less than	20g	25g
Cholesterol	Less than	300mg	300mg
Sodium	Less than	2,400mg	2,400mg
Total Carbohydrate		300g	375g
Dietary Fiber		25g	30g

Footnote

Quick Guide to % Daily Value

5% or less is Low
20% or more is High

acid. Look at the % Daily Value (%DV) column to see whether a food is high or low in nutrients. If you want to limit a nutrient (such as fat, saturated fat, cholesterol, sodium), try to choose foods with a lower %DV. If you want to consume more of a nutrient (such as calcium, other vitamins and minerals, fiber), try to choose foods with a higher %DV. As a guide, foods with 5%DV or less contribute a small amount of that nutrient to your eating pattern, while those with 20% or more contribute a large amount. Remember, Nutrition Facts serving sizes may differ from those used in the Food Guide Pyramid. For example, 2 ounces of dry macaroni yields about 1 cup cooked, or two (1/2 cup) Pyramid servings.

Use Of Dietary Supplements

Some people need a vitamin-mineral supplement to meet specific nutrient needs. For example, women who could become pregnant are advised to eat foods fortified with folic acid or to take a folic acid supplement in addition to consuming folate-rich foods to reduce the risk of some serious birth defects. Older adults and people with little exposure to sunlight may need a vitamin D supplement. People who seldom eat dairy products or other rich sources of calcium need a calcium supplement, and people who eat no animal foods need to take a vitamin B_{12} supplement. Sometimes vitamins or minerals are prescribed for meeting nutrient needs or for therapeutic purposes. For example, health care providers may advise pregnant women to take an iron supplement, and adults over age 50 to get their vitamin B_{12} from a supplement or from fortified foods.

Supplements of some nutrients, such as vitamin A and selenium, can be harmful if taken in large amounts. Because foods contain many substances that promote health, use the Food Guide Pyramid when choosing foods. Don't depend on supplements to meet your usual nutrient needs.

Dietary supplements include not only vitamins and minerals, but also amino acids, fiber, herbal products, and many other substances that are widely available. Herbal products usually provide a very small amount of vitamins and minerals. The value of herbal products for health is currently being studied. Standards for their purity, potency, and composition are being developed.

4. Choose A Variety Of Grains Daily, Especially Whole Grains

Foods made from grains (like wheat, rice, and oats) help form the foundation of a nutritious diet. They provide vitamins, minerals, carbohydrates (starch and dietary fiber), and other substances that are important for good health. Grain products are low in fat, unless fat is added in processing, in preparation, or at the table. Whole grains differ from refined grains in the amount of fiber and nutrients they provide, and different whole grain foods differ in nutrient content, so choose a variety of whole and enriched grains. Eating plenty of whole grains, such as whole wheat bread or oatmeal, as part of the healthful eating patterns described by these guidelines, may help protect you against many chronic diseases. Aim for at least 6 servings of grain products per day—more if you are an older child or teenager, an adult man, or an active woman—and include several servings of whole grain foods.

Why Choose Whole Grain Foods?

Vitamins, minerals, fiber, and other protective substances in whole grain foods contribute to the health benefits of whole grains. Refined grains are low in fiber and in the protective substances that accompany fiber. Eating plenty of fiber-containing foods, such as whole grains (and also many fruits and vegetables) promotes proper bowel function. The high fiber content of many whole grains may also help you to feel full with fewer calories. Fiber is best obtained from foods like whole grains, fruits, and vegetables rather than from fiber supplements for several reasons: there are many types of fiber, the composition of fiber is poorly understood, and other protective substances accompany fiber in foods. Use the Nutrition Facts Label to help choose grains that are rich in fiber and low in saturated fat and sodium.

Enriched Grains Are A New Source Of Folic Acid

Folic acid, a form of folate, is now added to all enriched grain products (thiamin, riboflavin, niacin, and iron have been added to enriched grains for many years). Folate is a B vitamin that reduces the risk of some serious types of birth defects when consumed before and during early pregnancy. Studies are underway to clarify whether it decreases risk for coronary heart disease, stroke, and certain types of cancer. Whole grain foods naturally contain some folate, but only a few (mainly ready-to-eat breakfast cereals) contain added folic acid as well. Read the ingredient label to find out if folic acid and other nutrients have been added, and check the Nutrition Facts Label to compare the nutrient content of foods like breakfast cereals.

5. Choose A Variety Of Fruits And Vegetables Daily

Fruits and vegetables are key parts of your daily diet. Eating plenty of fruits and vegetables of different kinds, as part of the healthful eating patterns described by these guidelines, may help protect you against many chronic diseases. It also promotes healthy bowel function. Fruits and vegetables provide essential vitamins and minerals, fiber, and other substances that are important for good health. Most people, including children, eat fewer servings of fruits and vegetables than are recommended. To promote your health, eat a variety of fruits and vegetables—at least 2 servings of fruits and 3 servings of vegetables—each day.

✔ Quick Tip

To increase your intake of whole grain foods, choose foods that name one of the following ingredients *first* on the label's ingredient list:

- brown rice
- oatmeal
- whole oats
- bulgur (cracked wheat)
- popcorn
- whole rye
- graham flour
- pearl barley
- whole wheat
- whole grain corn

Try some of these whole grain foods: whole wheat bread, whole grain ready-to-eat cereal, low-fat whole wheat crackers, oatmeal, whole wheat pasta, whole barley in soup, tabouli salad.

NOTE: "Wheat flour," "enriched flour," and "degerminated corn meal" are not whole grains.

Why Eat Plenty Of Different Fruits And Vegetables?

Different fruits and vegetables are rich in different nutrients. Some fruits and vegetables are excellent sources of carotenoids, including those which form vitamin A, while others may be rich in vitamin C, folate, or potassium. Fruits and vegetables, especially dry beans and peas, also contain fiber and other substances that are associated with good health. Dark-green leafy vegetables, deeply colored fruits, and dry beans and peas are especially rich in many nutrients. Most fruits and vegetables are naturally low in fat and calories and are filling. Some are high in fiber, and many are quick to prepare and easy to eat. Choose whole or cut-up fruits and vegetables rather than juices most often. Juices contain little or no fiber.

✔ Quick Tip

Find ways to include plenty of different fruits and vegetables in your meals and snacks.

- Buy wisely. Frozen or canned fruits and vegetables are sometimes best buys, and they are rich in nutrients. If fresh fruit is very ripe, buy only enough to use right away.

- Store properly to maintain quality. Refrigerate most fresh fruits (not bananas) and vegetables (not potatoes or tomatoes) for longer storage, and arrange them so you'll use up the ripest ones first.

- If you cut them up or open a can, cover and refrigerate afterward.

- Keep ready-to-eat raw vegetables handy in a clear container in the front of your refrigerator for snacks or meals-on-the-go.

- Keep a day's supply of fresh or dried fruit handy on the table or counter.

- Enjoy fruits as a naturally sweet end to a meal.

- When eating out, choose a variety of vegetables at a salad bar.

Aim For Variety

Try many colors and kinds. Choose any form: fresh, frozen, canned, dried, juices. All forms provide vitamins and minerals, and all provide fiber except for most juices—so choose fruits and vegetables most often.

Wash fresh fruits and vegetables thoroughly before using. If you buy prepared vegetables, check the Nutrition Facts Label to find choices that are low in saturated fat and sodium.

Try serving fruits and vegetables in new ways:

- raw vegetables with a low- or reduced-fat dip
- vegetables stir-fried in a small amount of vegetable oil
- fruits or vegetables mixed with other foods in salads, casseroles, soups, sauces (for example, add shredded vegetables when making meatloaf)

6. Keep Food Safe To Eat

Foods that are safe from harmful bacteria, viruses, parasites, and chemical contaminants are vital for healthful eating. *Safe* means that the food poses little risk of foodborne illness. Farmers, food producers, markets, food service establishments, and other food preparers have a role to keep food as safe as possible. However, we also need to keep and prepare foods safely in the home, and be alert when eating out. Follow the steps below to keep your food safe. Be very careful with perishable foods such as eggs, meats, poultry, fish, shellfish, milk products, and fresh fruits and vegetables. If you are at high risk of foodborne illness, be extra careful.

- *Clean.* Wash hands and surfaces often.
- *Separate.* Separate raw, cooked, and ready-to-eat foods while shopping, preparing, or storing.
- *Cook.* Cook foods to a safe temperature.
- *Chill.* Refrigerate perishable foods promptly.
- *Follow the label.* Read the label and follow safety instructions on the package such as "KEEP REFRIGERATED" and the "SAFE HANDLING INSTRUCTIONS."

- *Serve safely.* Keep hot foods hot (140° F or above) and cold foods cold (40° F or below).

- *When in doubt, throw it out.* If you aren't sure that food has been pre-pared, served, or stored safely, throw it out. You may not be able to make food safe if it has been handled in an unsafe manner.

7. Choose A Diet That Is Low In Saturated Fat And Cholesterol And Moderate In Total Fat

Fats supply energy and essential fatty acids, and they help absorb the fat-soluble vitamins A, D, E, and K, and carotenoids. You need some fat in the food you eat, but choose sensibly. Some kinds of fat, especially saturated fats, increase the risk for coronary heart disease by raising the blood choles-terol. In contrast, unsaturated fats (found mainly in vegetable oils) do not increase blood cholesterol. Fat intake in the United States as a pro-portion of total calories is lower than it was many years ago, but most people still eat too much saturated fat. Eating lots of fat of any type can provide excess calories.

Fats and Oils

- Choose vegetable oils rather than solid fats (meat and dairy fats, short-ening).

- If you need fewer calories, decrease the amount of fat you use in cook-ing and at the table.

Meat, Poultry, Fish, Shellfish, Eggs, Beans, and Nuts

- Choose 2 to 3 servings of fish, shell-fish, lean poultry, other lean meats, beans, or nuts daily. Trim fat from meat and take skin off poultry. Choose dry beans, peas, or lentils often.

✔ **Quick Tip**

Get most of your calo-ries from plant foods (grains, fruits, vegetables). If you eat foods high in saturated fat for a special occasion, return to foods that are low in satu-rated fat the next day.

- Limit your intake of high-fat processed meats such as bacon, sausages, salami, bologna, and other cold cuts. Try the lower fat varieties (check the Nutrition Facts Label).

- Limit your intake of liver and other organ meats. Use egg yolks and whole eggs in moderation. Use egg whites and egg substitutes freely when cooking since they contain no cholesterol and little or no fat.

Dairy Products

- Choose fat-free or low-fat milk, fat-free or low-fat yogurt, and low-fat cheese most often. Try switching from whole to fat-free or low-fat milk. This decreases the saturated fat and calories but keeps all other nutrients the same.

Prepared Foods

- Check the Nutrition Facts Label to see how much saturated fat and cholesterol are in a serving of prepared food. Choose foods lower in saturated fat and cholesterol.

Foods at Restaurants or Other Eating Establishments

- Choose fish or lean meats as suggested above. Limit ground meat and fatty processed meats, marbled steaks, and cheese.

- Limit your intake of foods with creamy sauces, and add little or no butter to your food.

- Choose fruits as desserts most often.

8. Choose Beverages And Foods To Moderate Your Intake Of Sugars

Sugars are carbohydrates and a source of energy (calories). Dietary carbohydrates also include the complex carbohydrates starch and dietary fiber. During digestion all carbohydrates except fiber break down into sugars. Sugars and starches occur naturally in many foods that also supply other nutrients. Examples of these foods include milk, fruits, some vegetables, breads, cereals, and grains.

Sugars And Tooth Decay

Foods containing sugars and starches can promote tooth decay. The amount of bacteria in your mouth and lack of exposure to fluorides also promote tooth decay. These bacteria use sugars and starches to produce the acid that causes tooth decay. The more often you eat foods that contain sugars and starches, and the longer these foods remain in your mouth before you brush your teeth, the greater your risk for tooth decay. Frequent eating or drinking sweet or starchy foods between meals is more likely to harm teeth than eating the same foods at meals and then brushing. Daily dental hygiene, including brushing with fluoride toothpaste and flossing, and adequate intake of fluorides will help prevent tooth decay.

Added Sugars

Added sugars are sugars and syrups added to foods in processing or preparation, not the naturally occurring sugars in foods like fruit or milk. The body cannot tell the difference between naturally occurring and added sugars because they are identical chemically. Foods containing added sugars provide calories, but may have few vitamins and minerals. In the United States, the number one source of added sugars is nondiet soft drinks (soda or pop). Sweets and candies, cakes and cookies, and fruit drinks and fruitades are also major sources of added sugars.

Intake of a lot of foods high in added sugars, like soft drinks, is of concern. Consuming excess calories from these foods may contribute to weight gain or lower consumption of more nutritious foods. Drink water to quench your thirst, and offer it to children.

Some foods with added sugars, like chocolate milk, presweetened cereals, and sweetened canned fruits, also are high in vitamins and minerals. These foods may provide extra calories along with the nutrients and are fine if you need the extra calories.

The Nutrition Facts Label gives the content of sugars from all sources (naturally occurring sugars plus added sugars, if any—see Table 11.1). You can use the Nutrition Facts Label to compare the amount of total sugars among similar products. To find out if sugars have been added, you also need to look at the food label ingredient list.

Table 11.1. Names for added sugars that appear on food labels.

A food is likely to be high in sugars if one of these names appears first or second in the ingredient list, or if several names are listed.

- Brown sugar
- Corn sweetener
- Corn syrup
- Dextrose
- Fructose
- Fruit juice con-centrate

- Glucose
- High-fructose corn syrup
- Honey
- Invert sugar
- Lactose

- Malt syrup
- Maltose
- Molasses
- Raw sugar
- Sucrose
- Syrup
- Table sugar

Sugar Substitutes

Sugar substitutes such as saccharin, aspartame, acesulfame potassium, and sucralose are extremely low in calories. Some people find them useful if they want a sweet taste without the calories. Some foods that contain sugar substitutes, however, still have calories. Unless you reduce the total calories you eat or increase your physical activity, using sugar substitutes will not cause you to lose weight.

Sugars And Other Health Issues

Behavior. Intake of sugars does not appear to affect children's behavior patterns or their ability to learn. Many scientific studies conclude that sugars do not cause hyperactivity in children.

Weight control. Foods that are high in sugars but low in essential nutrients primarily contribute calories to the diet. When you take in extra calories and don't offset them by increasing your physical activity, you will gain weight. As you aim for a healthy weight and fitness, keep an eye on portion size for all foods and beverages, not only those high in sugars.

9. Choose And Prepare Foods With Less Salt

Many people can reduce their chances of developing high blood pressure by consuming less salt. In the body, sodium—which you get mainly from salt—plays an essential role in regulating fluids and blood pressure. Many studies in diverse populations have shown that a high sodium intake is associated with higher blood pressure.

There is no way to tell who might develop high blood pressure from eating too much salt. However, consuming less salt or sodium is not harmful and can be recommended for the healthy, normal person.

At present, the firmest link between salt intake and health relates to blood pressure. High salt intake also increases the amount of calcium excreted in the urine. Eating less salt may decrease the loss of calcium from bone. Loss of too much calcium from bone increases the risk of osteoporosis and bone fractures.

Salt Is Found Mainly In Processed And Prepared Foods

Salt (sodium chloride) is the main source of sodium in foods. Only small amounts of salt occur naturally in foods. Most of the salt you eat comes from foods that have salt added during food processing or during preparation in a restaurant or at home. Some recipes include table salt or a salty broth or sauce, and some cooking styles call for adding a very salty seasoning such as soy sauce. Not all foods with added salt taste salty. Some people add salt or a salty seasoning to their food at the table. Your preference for salt may decrease if you gradually add smaller amounts of salt or salty seasonings to your food over a period of time.

Aim For A Moderate Sodium Intake

Most people consume too much salt, so moderate your salt intake. Healthy children and adults need to consume only small amounts of salt to meet their sodium needs—less than 1/4 teaspoon of salt daily. The Nutrition Facts Label lists a Daily Value of 2,400 mg of sodium per day. This is the amount of sodium in about 1 teaspoon of salt.

✔ Quick Tip

Ways to decrease your salt intake:

At The Store

- Choose fresh, plain frozen, or canned vegetables without added salt most often—they're low in salt.

- Choose fresh or frozen fish, shellfish, poultry, and meat most often. They are lower in salt than most canned and processed forms.

- Read the Nutrition Facts Label to compare the amount of sodium in processed foods—such as frozen dinners, packaged mixes, cereals, cheese, breads, soups, salad dressings, and sauces. The amount in different types and brands often varies widely.

- Look for labels that say "low-sodium." They contain 140 mg (about 5% of the Daily Value) or less of sodium per serving.

- Ask your grocer or supermarket to offer more low-sodium foods.

Cooking And Eating At Home

- If you salt foods in cooking or at the table, add small amounts. Learn to use spices and herbs, rather than salt, to enhance the flavor of food.

- Go easy on condiments such as soy sauce, ketchup, mustard, pickles, and olives—they can add a lot of salt to your food.

- Leave the salt shaker in a cupboard.

Eating Out

- Choose plain foods like grilled or roasted entrees, baked potatoes, and salad with oil and vinegar. Batter-fried foods tend to be high in salt, as do combination dishes like stews or pasta with sauce.

- Ask to have no salt added when the food is prepared.

Any Time

- Choose fruits and vegetables often.

- Drink water freely. It is usually very low in sodium. Check the label on bottled water for sodium content.

☞ Remember!!

- Aim for a healthy weight. If you are at a healthy weight, aim to avoid weight gain. If you are already overweight, first aim to prevent further weight gain, and then lose weight to improve your health.

- Get moving. Get regular physical activity to balance calories from the foods you eat. Consult your health care provider before starting a new vigorous physical activity plan if you have a chronic health problem, or if you are over 40 (men) or 50 (women).

- Keep in mind that even though heredity and the environment are important influences, your behaviors help determine your body weight.

- Build a healthy base: Use the Food Guide Pyramid to help make healthy food choices that you can enjoy.

- Build your eating pattern on a variety of plant foods, including whole grains, fruits, and vegetables. Also choose some low-fat dairy products and low-fat foods from the meat and beans group each day. It's fine to enjoy fats and sweets occasionally.

- Limit use of solid fats, such as butter, hard margarines, lard, and partially hydrogenated shortenings. Use vegetable oils as a substitute.

- Choose sensibly to limit your intake of beverages and foods that are high in added sugars. Take care not to let soft drinks or other sweets crowd out other foods you need to maintain health, such as low-fat milk or other good sources of calcium. Drink water often.

10. Adults Who Drink Alcoholic Beverages Should Do So In Moderation

Alcoholic beverages supply calories but few nutrients. Alcoholic beverages are harmful when consumed in excess, and some people should not drink at all. Excess alcohol alters judgment and can lead to dependency and a great many other serious health problems. Taking more than one drink per day for women or two drinks per day for men can raise the risk for motor vehicle crashes, other injuries, high blood pressure, stroke, violence, suicide, and certain types of cancer. Even one drink per day can slightly raise the risk of breast cancer. Alcohol consumption during pregnancy increases risk of birth defects. Too much alcohol may cause social and psychological problems, cirrhosis of the liver, inflammation of the pancreas, and damage to the brain and heart. Heavy drinkers also are at risk of malnutrition because alcohol contains calories that may substitute for those in nutritious foods. If adults choose to drink alcoholic beverages, they should consume them only in moderation and with meals to slow alcohol absorption.

♣ **It's A Fact!!**

Risk of alcohol abuse increases when drinking starts at an early age.

Who Should Not Drink?

Some people should not drink alcoholic beverages at all. These include:

- *Children and adolescents.*

- *Individuals of any age who cannot restrict their drinking to moderate levels.* This is a special concern for recovering alcoholics, problem drinkers, and people whose family members have alcohol problems.

- *Women who may become pregnant or who are pregnant.* A safe level of alcohol intake has not been established for women at any time during pregnancy, including the first few weeks. Major birth defects, including fetal alcohol syndrome, can be caused by heavy drinking by the pregnant mother. Other fetal alcohol effects may occur at lower levels.

- *Individuals who plan to drive, operate machinery, or take part in other activities that require attention, skill, or coordination.* Most people retain some alcohol in the blood up to 2 to 3 hours after a single drink.

- *Individuals taking prescription or over-the-counter medications that can interact with alcohol.* Alcohol alters the effectiveness or toxicity of many medications, and some medications may increase blood alcohol levels. If you take medications, ask your health care provider for advice about alcohol intake.

Chapter 12

Using The Food Guide Pyramid

What's In This Chapter For Me?

This chapter introduces you to The Food Guide Pyramid. The Pyramid illustrates the research-based food guidance system developed by the U.S. Department of Agriculture (USDA) and supported by the Department of Health and Human Services (DHHS). It goes beyond the "basic four food groups" to help you put the Dietary Guidelines into action.

The Pyramid is based on USDA's research on what foods Americans eat, what nutrients are in these foods, and how to make the best food choices for you.

The Pyramid and this chapter will help you choose what and how much to eat from each food group to get the nutrients you need and not too many calories, or too much fat, saturated fat, cholesterol, sugar, sodium, or alcohol.

The Pyramid focuses on fat because most American's diet are too high in fat. Following the Pyramid will help you keep your intake of total fat and saturated fat low. A diet low in fat will reduce your chances of getting certain diseases and help you maintain a healthy weight.

This chapter will also help you learn how to spot and control the sugars and salt in your diet, and make lower sugar and salt choices.

About This Chapter: The text in this chapter is from "The Food Guide Pyramid," U.S. Department of Agriculture (USDA) and U.S. Department of Health and Human Services (DHHS), April 19, 2000.

What's The Best Nutrition Advice?

The best nutrition advice is following the "Dietary Guidelines for Americans." By following the Dietary Guidelines, you can enjoy better health and reduce your chances of getting certain diseases. These Guidelines, developed jointly by USDA and DHHS, are the best, most up-to-date advice from nutrition scientists and are the basis of Federal nutrition policy. (For more information about the Dietary Guidelines, see Chapter 11).

What Is The Food Guide Pyramid?

The Pyramid is an outline of what to eat each day. It's not a rigid prescription, but a general guide that lets you choose a healthful diet that's right for you.

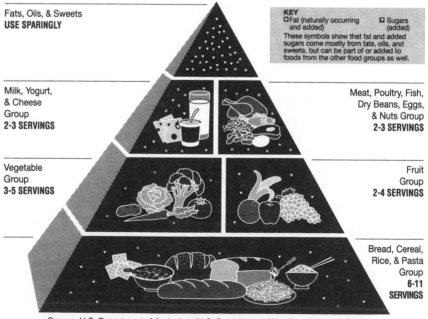

Fats, Oils, & Sweets
USE SPARINGLY

KEY
□ Fat (naturally occurring   ▨ Sugars
and added)   (added)
These symbols show that fat and added sugars come mostly from fats, oils, and sweets, but can be part of or added to foods from the other food groups as well.

Milk, Yogurt,
& Cheese
Group
2-3 SERVINGS

Meat, Poultry, Fish,
Dry Beans, Eggs,
& Nuts Group
2-3 SERVINGS

Vegetable
Group
3-5 SERVINGS

Fruit
Group
2-4 SERVINGS

Bread, Cereal,
Rice, & Pasta
Group
**6-11
SERVINGS**

Source: U.S. Department of Agriculture/U.S. Department of Health and Human Services

Figure 12.1. The Food Guide Pyramid. Source: U.S. Department of Agriculture (USDA) and the U.S. Department of Health and Human Services (DHHS).

The Pyramid calls for eating a variety of foods to get the nutrients you need and at the same time the right amount of calories to maintain or improve your weight.

The Pyramid also focuses on fat because most Americans diets are too high in fat, especially saturated fat.

Looking At The Pieces Of The Pyramid

The Food Guide Pyramid emphasizes foods from the five major food groups shown in the three lower sections of the Pyramid. Each of these food groups provides some, but not all, of the nutrients you need. Foods in one group can't replace those in another. No one food group is more important than another—for good health, you need them all.

The small tip of the Pyramid shows fats, oils, and sweets. These are foods such as salad dressings and oils, cream, butter, margarine, sugars, soft drinks, candies, and sweet desserts. These foods provide calories and little else nutritionally. Most people should use them sparingly.

On the next level of the Food Guide Pyramid are two groups of foods that come mostly from animals: milk, yogurt, cheese; and meat, poultry, fish, dry beans, eggs, and nuts. These foods are for protein, calcium, iron, and zinc.

The next level includes foods that come from plants—vegetables and fruits. Most people need to eat more of these foods for the vitamins, minerals, and fiber they supply.

At the base of the Food Guide Pyramid are breads, cereals, rice, and pasta—all foods from grains. You need the servings of these foods each day.

✎ Weird Words

Carbohydrates: Starches; an important source of energy, especially in low-fat diets.

Calories: Units that measure the energy the body gets from food. Your body needs calories as "fuel" to perform all of its functions such as breathing, circulating the blood, and physical activity.

A Closer Look At Fat And Added Sugars

As you can see, fat and sugars are concentrated in foods from the Pyramid tip—fats, oils, and sweets. These foods supply calories, but little or no vitamins and minerals. By using these foods sparingly, you can have a diet that supplies needed vitamins and minerals without excess calories.

Some fat or sugar symbols are shown in the food groups. That's to remind you that some food choices in these food groups can also be high in fat or added sugars. When choosing foods for a healthful diet, consider that fat and added sugars in your choices from the food groups, as well as the fats, oils, and sweets from the Pyramid tip.

Fat

In general, foods that come from animals (milk and meat groups) are naturally higher in fat than foods that come from plants. But there are many low-fat dairy and lean meat choices available, and these foods can be prepared in ways that lower fat.

Fruits, vegetables, and grain products are naturally low in fat. But many popular items are prepared with fat, like french-fried potatoes, or croissants, making them higher fat choices.

♣ It's A Fact!!

Many popular items are prepared with fat making them higher fat choices. For example:

- One Baked Potato
  Calories: 120
  Fat: Trace

- 14 French Fries
  Calories: 225
  Fat: 11 grams

Added Sugars

These symbols represent sugars added to foods in processing or at the table, not the sugars found naturally in fruits and milk. It's the added sugars that provide calories with few vitamins and minerals.

Most of the added sugars in the typical American diet come from foods in the Pyramid tip—soft drinks, candy, jams, jellies, syrups, and table sugar we add to foods like coffee or cereal.

Added sugars in the food groups come from foods such as ice cream, sweetened yogurt, chocolate milk, canned or frozen fruit with heavy syrup, an sweetened bakery products like cakes and cookies.

✔ Quick Tip

To reduce your consumption of fat and sugar:

- Choose lower fat foods from the food groups most often.
- Go easy on fats and sugars added to foods in cooking or at the table— butter, margarine, gravy, salad dressing, sugar, and jelly.
- Choose fewer foods that are high in sugars—candy, sweet desserts, and soft drinks.

How To Make The Pyramid Work For You

How Many Servings Are Right For Me?

The Pyramid shows a range of servings for each major food group. The number of servings that are right for you depends on how many calories you need, which in turn depends on your age, sex, size, and how active you are. Almost everyone should have at least the lowest number of servings in the ranges.

The calorie level suggestions are based on recommendations of the National Academy of Sciences and on calorie intakes reported by people in national food consumption surveys.

Now, take a look at Table 12.1. It tells you how many servings you need for your calorie level. For example, if you are an active woman who needs about 2,200 calories a day, 9 servings of breads, cereals, rice, or pasta would be right for you. You'd also want to eat about 6 ounces of meat or alternates per day. Keep total fat (fat in the foods you choose as well as fat used in cooking or added at the table) to about 73 grams per day.

If you are between calorie categories, estimate servings. For example, some less active women may need only 2,000 calories to maintain a healthy weight. At that calorie level, 8 servings from the grain group would be about right.

Table 12.1. Sample Diets For A Day At 3 Calorie Levels

	Lower[1] about 1,600	Moderate[2] about 2,200	Higher[3] about 2,800
Grain Group # of Servings	6	9	11
Vegetable Group # of Servings	3	4	5
Fruit Group # of Servings	2	3	4
Milk Group # of Servings*	2-3	2-3	2-3
Meat Group # of ounces	5	6	7
Total Fat # of grams	53	73	93
Total Added Sugars # of teaspoons	6	12	18

*Women who are pregnant or breastfeeding, teenagers, and young adults to age 24 need 3 servings.

Examples of people in each calorie group:

1. *Children ages 2 to 6 years, women, some older adults*

2. *Older children, teen girls, active women, most men*

3. *Teen boys, active men*

What Is A Serving?

The amount of food that counts as a serving is listed in Table 12.2. If you eat a larger portion, count it as more than one serving. For example, 1/2 cup of cooked pasta counts as one serving in the bread, cereal, rice, and pasta group. If you eat 1 cup of pasta, that would be two servings. If you eat a smaller portion, count it as part of a serving.

Isn't 6 To 11 Servings Of Breads And Cereals A Lot?

It may sound like a lot, but it's really not. For example, a slice of bread is one serving, so a sandwich for lunch would equal two servings. A small bowl of cereal and one slice of toast for breakfast are two more servings. And it you have a cup of rice or pasta at dinner, that's two more servings. A snack of 3 or 4 small plain crackers adds yet another serving. So now you've had 7 servings. It adds up quicker than you think!

Do I Need To Measure Servings?

No. Use servings only as a general guide. For mixed foods, do the best you can to estimate the food group servings of the main ingredients. For example, a generous serving of pizza would count in the grain group (crust), the milk group (cheese), and the vegetable group (tomato); a helping of beef stew would count in the meat group and the vegetable group. Both have some fat—fat in the cheese on the pizza and in the gravy form the stew, if it's made from meat drippings.

✔ Quick Tip

You can figure the number of grams of fat that provide 30% of calories in your daily diet as follow:

A. Multiply your total day's calories by 0.30 to get your calories from fat per day. Example: 2,200 calories x 0.30 = 660 calories from fat.

B. Divide calories from fat per day by 9 (each gram of fat has 9 calories) to get grams of fat per day. Example: 660 calories from fat ÷ 9 = 73 grams of fat.

Table 12.2. What Counts As A Serving?

Bread, Cereal, Rice, and Pasta Group (Grains Group)—whole grain and refined
- 1 slice of bread
- About 1 cup of ready-to-eat cereal
- 1/2 cup of cooked cereal, rice, or pasta

Vegetable Group
- 1 cup of raw leafy vegetables
- 1/2 cup of other vegetables—cooked or raw
- 3/4 cup of vegetable juice

Fruit Group
- 1 medium apple, banana, orange, pear
- 1/2 cup of chopped, cooked, or canned fruit
- 3/4 cup of fruit juice

Milk, Yogurt, and Cheese Group (Milk Group)*
- 1 cup of milk** or yogurt**
- 1 1/2 ounces of natural cheese** (such as Cheddar)
- 2 ounces of processed cheese** (such as American)

Meat, Poultry, Fish, Dry Beans, Eggs, and Nuts Group (Meat and Beans Group)
- 2–3 ounces of cooked lean meat, poultry, or fish
- 1/2 cup of cooked dry beans# or 1/2 cup of tofu counts as 1 ounce of lean meat
- 2 1/2-ounce soyburger or 1 egg counts as 1 ounce of lean meat
- 2 tablespoons of peanut butter or 1/3 cup of nuts counts as 1 ounce of meat

NOTE: Many of the serving sizes given above are smaller than those on the Nutrition Facts Label. For example, 1 serving of cooked cereal, rice, or pasta is 1 cup for the label but only 1/2 cup for the Pyramid.

* This includes lactose-free and lactose-reduced milk products. One cup of soy-based beverage with added calcium is an option for those who prefer a non-dairy source of calcium.

** Choose fat-free or reduced-fat dairy products most often.

 # Dry beans, peas, and lentils can be counted as servings in either the meat and beans group or the vegetable group. As a vegetable, 1/2 cup of cooked, dry beans counts as 1 serving. As a meat substitute, 1 cup of cooked, dry beans counts as 1 serving (2 ounces of meat).

Source: Nutrition and Your Health: Dietary Guidelines for Americans, Fifth Edition, *2000, Home and Garden Bulletin No. 232, United States Department of Agriculture (USDA).*

What If I Want To Lose Or Gain Weight?

The best and simplest way to lose weight is to increase your physical activity and reduce the fat and sugars in your diet.

But be sure to eat at least the lowest number of servings from the five major food groups in the Food Guide Pyramid. You need them for the vitamins, minerals, carbohydrates, and protein they provide. Just try to pick the lowest fat choices from the food groups.

To gain weight, increase the amounts of foods you eat from all of the food groups. If you have lost weight unexpectedly, see your doctor.

Fats

How Much Fat Can I Have?

It depends on your calorie needs. *The Dietary Guidelines* recommend that Americans limit fat in their diets to 30 percent of calories. This amounts to 53 grams of fat in a 1,600-calorie diet, 73 grams of fat in a 2,200-calorie diet, and 93 grams of fat in a 2,800-calorie diet.

You will get up to half this fat even if you pick the lowest fat choice from each good group and add no fat to your foods in preparation or at the table.

You decide how to use the additional fat in your daily diet. You may want to have foods from the five major food groups that are higher in fat—such as whole milk instead of skim milk. Or you may want to use it in cooking or at the table in the form of spreads, dressings, or toppings.

How To Check Your Diet For Fat

If you want to be sure you have a low-fat diet, you can count the grams of fat in your day's food choices using the Pyramid Food Choices Chart, and compare them to the number of grams of fat suggested for you calorie level.

You don't need to count fat grams every day, but doing a fat checkup once in awhile will help keep you on the right track. If you find you are eating too much fat, choose lower fat foods more often.

♣ It's A Fact!!

The number of calories you need depends on your age, sex, size, and how active you are. Here are some general guidelines for adults and teens:

- 1,600 calories is about right for many sedentary women and some older adults.

- 2,200 calories is about right for most children, teenage girls, active women, and many sedentary men. Women who are pregnant or breastfeeding may need somewhat more.

- 2,800 calories is about right for teenage boys, many active men, and some very active women.

Are Some Types Of Fat Worse Than Others?

Yes. Eating too much saturated fat raises blood cholesterol levels in many people, increasing their risk for heart disease. The Dietary Guidelines recommend limiting saturated fat to less than 10 percent of calories, or about on-third of total fat intake.

All fats in foods are mixtures of three types of fatty acids—saturated, monounsaturated, and polyunsaturated.

Saturated fats are found in largest amounts in fats from meat and dairy product and in some vegetables fats such as coconut, palm, and palm kernel oils.

Monounsaturated fats are found mainly in olive, peanut, and canola oils.

Polyunsaturated fats are found mainly in safflower, sunflower, corn, soybean, and cottonseed oils and some fish.

How Do I Avoid Too Much Saturated Fat?

Follow the Food Guide Pyramid, keeping your total fat within recommended. Choose fat from a variety of food sources, but mostly from those foods that are higher in polyunsaturated or monounsaturated fat.

Cholesterol

What About Cholesterol?

Cholesterol and fat are not the same thing.

Cholesterol is a fat-like substance present in all animal foods—meat, poultry, fish, milk and milk products, and egg yolks. Both the lean and fat of meat and the meat and skin of poultry contain cholesterol. In milk products, cholesterol is mostly in the fat, so lower fat products contain less cholesterol. Egg yolks and organ meats, like liver, are high in cholesterol. Plant foods do not contain cholesterol.

Dietary cholesterol, as well as saturated fat, raises blood cholesterol levels in many people, increasing their risk for heart disease. Some health authorities recommend that dietary cholesterol be limited to an average of 300 mg or less per day. To keep dietary cholesterol to this level, follow the Food Guide Pyramid, keeping your total fat to the amount that's right for you.

It's not necessary to eliminate all foods that are high in cholesterol. You can have three to four egg yolks a week, counting those used as ingredients in custards and baked products. Use lower fat dairy products often and occasionally include dry beans and peas in place of meat.

✔ Quick Tip

Here are some selection tips for lowing your intake of saturated fat:

- Use lean meats and skim or low-fat dairy products.

- Use unsaturated vegetable oils and margarines that list a liquid vegetable oil as first ingredient on the label.

- Read nutrition and ingredient labels on food packages to check the kinds and amounts of fat they contain.

- Limit use of products that contain a large amount of saturated fats. Examples are nondairy creamers and rich baked products such as pie crusts and other pastries, cakes, and cookies.

Sugars

Choosing a diet low in fat is a concern for everyone; choosing one low in sugars is also important for people who have low calorie needs. Sugars include white sugar, brown sugar, raw sugar, corn syrup, honey, and molasses; these supply calories and little else nutritionally.

To avoid getting too many calories from sugars, try to limit your added sugars to 6 teaspoons a day if you eat about 1,600 calories, 12 teaspoons at 2,200 calories, or 18 teaspoons at 2,800 calories. These amounts are intended to be averages over time.

Table 12.3. Where are the added sugars?

Food Groups	Added Sugars (teaspoons)	Food Groups	Added Sugars (teaspoons)
Bread, Cereal, Rice, and Pasta		*Milk, Yogurt, and Cheese*	
Bread, 1 slice	0	Milk, plain, 1 cup	0
Muffin, 1 medium	1	Chocolate milk, 2 percent, 1 cup	3
Cookies, 2 medium	1	Lowfat yogurt, plain, 8 oz.	0
Danish pasty, 1 medium	1	Lowfat, yogurt, flavored, 8 oz.	5
Doughnut, 1 medium	2	Lowfat yogurt, fruit, 8 oz.	7
Ready-to-eat cereal, sweetened, 1 oz.	*	Ice Cream, ice milk, frozen yogurt 1/2 cup	3
Pound cake, no-fat, 1 oz.	2	Chocolate shake, 10 fl. oz	9
Angelfood cake, 1/12 tube cake	5		
Cake, frosted, 1/16 average	6	*Other*	
Pie, fruit, 2 crust, 1/6 8" pie	6	Sugar, jam, or jelly, 1 tsp.	1
		Syrup or honey, 1 tbsp.	3
Fruit		Chocolate bar, 1 oz.	3
Fruit, canned in juice, 1/2 cup	0	Fruit sorbet, 1/2 cup	3
Fruit, canned in light syrup, 1/2 cup	2	Gelatin dessert, 1/2 cup	4
Fruit, canned in heavy syrup, 1/2 cup	4	Sherbet, 1/2 cup	5
		Cola, 12 fl. oz.	9
		Fruit drink, ade, 12 fl. oz.	12

* Check product label.
Note: 4 grams of sugar = 1 teaspoon

Added sugars are in foods like candy and soft drinks, as well as jams, jellies, and sugars you add at the table. Some added sugars are also in foods from the food groups, such as fruit canned in heavy syrup and chocolate milk. Table 12.3 shows the approximate amount of sugars in some popular foods.

Salt And Sodium
Do I Have To Give Up Salt?

No. But most people eat more than they need. Some health authorities say that sodium intake should not be more than 2,400 mg. Nutrition labels also list a Daily Value (upper limit) of 2,400 mg per day of sodium. Much of the sodium in people's diets comes from salt they add while cooking and at the table. (One teaspoon of salt provides about 2,000 mg of sodium.)

Go easy on salt and foods that are high in sodium, including cured meats, luncheon meats, and many cheeses, most canned soups and vegetables, and soy sauce. Look for lower salt and no-salt-added versions of these products at your supermarket.

Table 12.4 will give you an idea of the amount of sodium in different types of foods. Information on food labels can also help you make food choices to keep sodium moderate.

The Food Groups
Why Are Breads, Cereals, Rice, And Pasta Important?

These foods provide complex carbohydrates (starches), which are an important source of energy, especially in low-fat diets.

They also provide vitamins, minerals, and fiber. The Food Guide Pyramid suggests 6 to 11 servings of these foods a day.

Aren't Starchy Foods Fattening?

No. It's what you add to these foods or cook with them that adds most of the calories. For example: margarine or butter on bread, cream or cheese sauces on pasta, and the sugar and fat used with the flour in making cookies.

Table 12.4. Where's the salt?

Food Groups	Sodium, mg
Bread, Cereal, Rice, and Pasta	
Cooked cereal, rice, pasta, unsalted, 1/2 cup	Trace
Ready-to-eat cereal, 1 oz.	100-360
Bread, 1 slice	110-175
Popcorn, salted, 1 oz.	100-460
Pretzels, salted, 1 oz.	130-880
Vegetables	
Vegetables, fresh or frozen, cooked without salt, 1/2 cup	Less than 70
Vegetables, canned or frozen with sauce, 1/2 cup	140-460
Tomato juice, canned, 3/4 cup	660
Vegetable soup, canned, 1 cup	820
Fruit	
Fruit, fresh, frozen, canned, 1/2 cup	Trace
Milk, Yogurt, and Cheese	
Milk, 1 cup	120
Yogurt, 8 oz.	160
Natural cheeses, 1-1/2 oz.	110-450
Process cheeses, 2 oz.	800
Meat, Poultry, Fish, Dry Beans, Eggs, and Nuts	
Fresh meat, poultry, fish, 3 oz.	Less than 90
Tuna, canned, water pack, 3 oz.	300
Bologna, 2 oz.	580
Ham, lean, roasted, 3 oz.	1,020
Peanuts, roasted in oil, salted, 1 oz.	120

Why Are Vegetables Important?

Vegetables provide vitamins, such as vitamins A and C, and folate, and minerals, such as iron and magnesium. They are naturally low in fat and also provide fiber. The Food Guide Pyramid suggests 3 to 5 servings of these foods a day.

✔ **Quick Tip**

Here are some selection tips for breads, cereals, rice, and pasta:

- To get the fiber you need, choose several servings a day of foods made from whole grains, such as whole-wheat bread and whole-grain cereals.

- Choose most often foods that are made with little fat or sugars. These include bread, English muffins, rice, and pasta.

- Baked goods made from flour, such as cakes, cookies, croissants, and pastries, count as part of this food group, but they are high in fat and sugars.

- Go easy on the fat and sugars you add as spreads, seasonings, or toppings.

- When preparing pasta, stuffing, and sauce from packaged mixes, use only half the butter or margarine suggested; if milk or cream is called for, use low-fat milk.

✔ **Quick Tip**

Here are some selection tips for choosing vegetables:

- Different types of vegetables provide different nutrients. For variety eat: dark-green leafy vegetables (spinach, romaine lettuce, broccoli); deep-yellow vegetables (carrots, sweet potatoes); starchy vegetables (potatoes, corn, peas); legumes (navy, pinto, and kidney beans, chickpeas); other vegetables (lettuce, tomatoes, onions, green beans)

- Include dark-green leafy vegetables and legumes several times a week—they are especially good sources of vitamins and minerals. Legumes also provide protein and can be used in place of meat.

- Go easy of the fat you add to vegetables at the table or during cooking. Added spreads or toppings, such as butter, mayonnaise, and salad dressing, count as fat.

- Use low-fat salad dressing.

Why Are Fruits Important?

Fruit and fruit juices provide important amounts of vitamins A and C and potassium. They are low in fat and sodium. The Food Guide Pyramid suggests 2 to 4 servings of fruits a day.

Why Are Meat, Poultry, Fish, And Other Foods In This Group Important?

Meat, poultry, and fish supply protein, B vitamins, iron, and zinc. The other foods in this group—dry beans, eggs, and nuts—are similar to meats in providing protein and most vitamins and minerals. The Food Guide Pyramid suggests 2 to 3 servings each day of foods from this group. The total amount of these servings should be the equivalent of 5 to 7 ounces of cooked lean meat, poultry, or fish per day.

> ✔ Quick Tip
>
> Here are some selection tips for choosing fruits:
>
> - Choose fresh fruits, fruit juices, and frozen, canned, or dried fruit. Pass up fruit canned or frozen in heavy syrups and sweetened fruit juices unless you have calories to spare.
>
> - Eat whole fruits often— they are higher in fiber than fruit juices.
>
> - Have citrus fruits, melon, and berries regularly. They are rich in vitamin C.
>
> - Count only 100 percent fruit juice as fruit. Punches, ades, and most fruit "drinks" contain only a little juice and lots of added sugars. Grape and orange sodas don't count as fruit juice.

What Counts As A Serving?

- Count 2-3 ounces of cooked lean meat, poultry, or fish as a serving. A 3-ounce piece of meat is about the size of an average hamburger, or the amount of meat on a medium chicken breast half.

- For other foods in this group, count 1/2 cup of cooked dry beans or 1 egg as 1 ounce of lean meat. 2 tablespoons of peanut butter or 1/3 cup of nuts count as 1 ounce of meat (about 1/3 serving).

Counting to see if you have an equivalent of 5-7 ounces of cooked lean meat a day is tricky. Portions sizes vary with the type of food and meal. For example, 6 ounces might come from:

- 1 egg (count as 1 oz. of lean meat) for breakfast;
- 2 oz. of sliced turkey in a sandwich at lunch; and
- a 3 oz. cooked lean hamburger for dinner.

Lean Choices

- Beef Roasts/Steaks: Round; Loin; Sirloin; Chuck Arm
- Pork Roasts/Chops: Tenderloin; Center Loin; Ham
- Veal: All cuts except ground
- Lamb Roasts/Chops: Leg; Loin; Fore Shanks
- Chicken and Turkey: Light and dark meat, without the skin
- Fish and shellfish: Most are low in fat; those marinated or canned in oil are higher

✔ Quick Tip

Here are some selection tips for choosing meat, poultry, fish, and other foods in the same group:

- Choose lean meat, poultry without skin, fish, and dry beans and peas often. They are the choices lowest in fat.

- Prepare meats in low-fat ways: trim away all the fat you can see; broil, roast, or boil these foods, instead of frying them.

- Go easy of egg yolk; they are high in cholesterol. Use only one yolk per person in egg dishes. Make larger portions by adding extra egg whites.

- Nuts and seeds are high in fat, so eat them in moderation.

Why Are Milk Products Important?

Milk products provide protein, vitamins, and minerals. Milk, yogurt, and cheese are the best source of calcium. The Food Guide Pyramid suggests 2 to 3 servings of milk, yogurt, and cheese a day—2 for most people, and 3 for women who are pregnant or breastfeeding, teenagers, and young adults to age 24.

The Pyramid Food Choices

Table 12.5 lists commonly used foods in each food group and the amount of fat in each. Only a few of the thousands of foods we eat are listed. However, they will give you an idea of foods from each food group that are higher and lower in fat.

Table 12.5. The fat content of selected foods. The Food Guide Pyramid symbol (») next to the food items means that food is one of the lowest fat choices you can make in that food group. You can use the food label to count fat in specific foods. Many food labels list the grams of fat in a serving.

For this amount of food...	number of servings	count this many grams of fat
Bread, Cereal, Rice, and Pasta Group, *Eat, 6 to 11 servings daily*		
»Bread, 1 slice	1	1
»Hamburger roll, bagel, English muffin, 1	2	2
Tortilla, 1	1	3
»Rice, pasta, cooked, 1/2 cup	1	Trace
Plain crackers, small, 3-4	1	3
Breakfast cereal, 1 oz.	1	*
Pancakes, 4" diameter, 2	2	3
Croissant, 1 large (2 oz.)	2	12
Doughnut, 1 medium (2 oz.)	2	11
Danish, 1 medium (2 oz.)	2	13
Cake, frosted, 1/16 average	1	13
Cookies, 2 medium	1	4
Pie, fruit, 2-crust, 1/6 8" pie	2	19
Vegetable Group, *Eat 3 to 5 servings daily*		
»Vegetables, cooked 1/2 cup	1	Trace
»Vegetables, leafy, raw 1 cup	1	Trace
»Vegetables, nonleafy, raw, chopped 1/2 cup	1	Trace
Potatoes, scalloped, 1/2 cup	1	4
Potato salad, 1/2 cup	1	8
French fries, 10	1	8
Fruit Group, *Eat 2 to 4 servings daily*		
»Whole fruit: medium apple, orange, banana	1	Trace
»Fruit, raw or canned, 1/2 cup	1	Trace
»Fruit juice, unsweetened, 3/4 cup	1	Trace
Avocado, 1/4 whole	1	9

» This symbol means that the item listed is one of the lowest fat choices in the group.
* Check product label

For this amount of food...	number of servings	count this many grams of fat
Milk, Yogurt, and Cheese Group, Eat 2 to 3 servings daily		
»Skim milk, 1 cup	1	Trace
»Nonfat yogurt, plain, 8 oz.	1	Trace
Low-fat milk, 2 percent, 1 cup	1	5
Whole milk, 1 cup	1	8
Chocolate milk, 2 percent, 1 cup	1	5
Low-fat yogurt, plain, 8 oz.	1	4
Low-fat yogurt, fruit, 8 oz.	1	3
Natural cheddar cheese, 1-1/2 oz.	1	14
Process cheese, 2 oz.	1	18
Mozzarella, part skim, 1/2 cup	1	7
Ricotta, part skim, 1/2 cup	1	10
Cottage cheese, 4 percent fat, 1/2 cup	1/4	5
Ice cream, 1/2 cup	1/3	7
Ice milk, 1/2 cup	1/3	3
Frozen yogurt, 1/2 cup	1/2	2
Meat, Poultry, Fish, Dry Beans, Eggs, and Nuts Group, Eat 5 to 7 oz. daily		
»Lean meat, poultry, fish, cooked	3 oz.	6
Ground beef, lean, cooked	3 oz.	16
Chicken, with skin, fried	3 oz.	13
Bologna, 2 slices	1 oz.	16
Egg, 1	1 oz.	5
»Dry beans and peas, cooked, 1/2 cup	1 oz.	Trace
Peanut butter, 2 tbsp.	1 oz.	16
Nuts, 1/3 cup	1 oz.	22
Fats, Oil, and Sweets, Use sparingly		
Butter, margarine, 1 tsp.	—	4
Mayonnaise, 1 tbsp.	—	11
Salad dressing, 1 tbsp.	—	7
Reduced calorie salad dressing, 1 tbsp.	—	*
Sour cream, 2 tbsp.	—	6
Cream cheese, 1 oz.	—	10
Sugar, jam, jelly, 1 tsp.	—	0
Cola, 12 fl. oz.	—	0
Fruit drink, ade, 12 fl. oz.	—	0
Chocolate bar, 1 oz.	—	9
Sherbet, 1/2 cup	—	2
Fruit sorbet, 1/2 cup	—	0
Gelatin dessert, 1/2 cup	—	0

✔ **Quick Tip**

Here are some selection tips for choosing milk products:

- Choose skim milk and nonfat yogurt often. They are lowest in fat.

- 1-1/2 to 2 ounces of cheese and 8 ounces of yogurt count as a serving from this group because they supply the same amount of calcium as 1 cup of milk.

- Cottage cheese is lower in calcium than most cheeses. One cup of cottage cheese counts as only 1/2 serving of milk.

- Go easy on high fat cheese and ice cream. They can add a lot of fat (especially saturated fat) to your diet.

- Choose "part skim" or low-fat cheeses when available and lower fat milk desserts, like ice milk or frozen yogurt.

How Much Is A Gram Of Fat?

To help you visualize how much fat is in foods, keep in mind that 1 teaspoon (1 pat) of butter has 4 grams of fat.

How To Rate Your Diet

You may want to rate you diet for a few days. Follow these four steps.

1. Jot down everything you ate yesterday for meals and snacks.

2. Write down the number of grams of fat in each food you list.

    - Use the Pyramid Food Choices Chart to get an idea of the number of grams of fat to count for the foods you ate.

    - Use nutrition labels on packaged foods you ate to find out the grams of fat they contained.

3. Answer these questions:

    - Did you have the number of servings from the five major food groups that are right for you?

- Add up your grams of fat listed in Step 2. Did you have more fat than the amount right for you?

- Do you need to watch the amount of added sugars you eat?

4. Decide what changes you can make for a healthier diet. Start by making small changes, like switching to low-fat salad dressings or adding an extra serving of vegetables. Make additional changes gradually until healthy eating becomes a habit.

☞ Remember!!

The Food Guide Pyramid illustrates the research-based food guidance system developed by USDA and supported by the Department of Health and Human Services (DHHS). It goes beyond the "basic four food groups" to help you put the Dietary Guidelines into action.

The Pyramid is based on USDA's research on what foods Americans eat, what nutrients are in these foods, and how to make the best food choices for you.

Following the Pyramid will help you keep your intake of total fat and saturated fat low. A diet low in fat will reduce your chances of getting certain diseases and help you maintain a healthy weight.

For more information about the Dietary Guidelines, contact USDA's Center for Nutrition Policy and Promotion. The address is:

U.S. Department of Agriculture
Center for Nutrition Policy and Promotion
Suite 200, North Lobby
1120 20th St., NW
Washington, DC 20036-3406
(202) 418-2312
http://www.usda.gov/cnpp

Chapter 13

Special Dietary Guidelines For Teenage Mothers

There are Recommended Dietary Allowances, or RDAs, for teenagers and for women nursing a baby. But should there be special nutritional guidelines for teenage mothers who are nursing? Some preliminary research suggests it might be a good idea.

Pediatrician Kathleen Motil, who is with the Agricultural Research Service's Children's Nutrition Research Center in Houston, Texas, compared the milk production of 22 mothers—half teens, half adults. The nutrient compositions were similar, but the teens produced 37 to 54 percent less milk than adults. Motil's findings were published in the *Journal of Adolescent Health*.

Motil said the differences between adult and teen milk production remained statistically significant, even after she adjusted the data for differences in feeding time and daily nursing frequency. Why should the milk volume be different? Motil has a theory.

"Our preliminary observations suggest that teenage mothers are facing a dual metabolic challenge," said Motil. "It may be they are still growing, themselves, which may cause an extra nutritional demand."

About This Chapter: The text in this chapter is from "Special Dietary Guidelines for Teenage Mothers," by Jill Lee, in the March 1998 issue of *Agricultural Research* magazine, produced by the U. S. Department of Agriculture.

Motil and her colleagues wanted to find out more about teen nutrition during lactation. They measured body composition, dietary intakes, and milk production. The participants: 24 teenage mothers, half of whom breastfed their infants. Eleven additional teens who had never been pregnant served as a control group. Barbara Kertz, patient service coordinator at the nutrition research center, organized the study.

Preliminary findings suggest that teenagers who nurse their infants continue to add muscle mass to their bodies, indicating ongoing growth.

"We found that nursing teens consumed more energy (calories), protein, and vitamin B6 than teen mothers who bottle-fed or teens who never had children," says Kertz. "They were taking in 23 percent more calories and vitamin B6 and 40 percent more protein." The teens' intake returned to regular levels after weaning. This research team also included nutritionist Corinne Montandon, who helped the girls keep a food journal to track the amounts and kinds of foods they ate. Montandon reviewed the journals for accuracy and sometimes provided a little advice. She cautioned one mother, for example, against trying to crash diet her way back to a pre-pregnancy figure.

❖ It's A Fact!!

According to the results of one study, teens who were nursing infants produced 37 to 54 percent less milk than adults who were nursing infants.

Encouraging Breastfeeding

Knowing about teenagers' nutritional demands during breastfeeding fits into a bigger plan of encouraging all mothers to breastfeed—regardless of age. In fact, USDA's Food and Nutrition Service (FNS) has started a nationwide campaign to encourage breastfeeding.

The number of U.S. teenagers becoming pregnant has been declining, but many groups estimate half a million girls under 20 do give birth annually. For those who choose to raise their infants, breastfeeding can offer advantages such as protection against a broad range of infections and enhanced bonding.

Teenagers are less likely to chose breastfeeding than adults, however. During an FNS focus group on breastfeeding, women of all ages cited embarrassment and lack of family support as barriers to breastfeeding.

But teens face special problems, according to a survey by Alain Joffe, M.D., of the Department of Pediatrics at Johns Hopkins University Hospital. Joffe has studied breastfeeding among 250 inner city teens in Baltimore, Maryland. Susan Radius, a sociologist at nearby Towson University, was a co-author.

The researchers found teenage mothers who returned to high school had a hard time working nursing into their schedule.

Joffe said in his survey the best indicator of whether a teen would breastfeed successfully was having a breastfeeding mentor. That person could be her mother, aunt, or other older friend who had breastfed successfully and could provide advice.

He added that for teens to accept breastfeeding they must know the benefits and feel confident about ways of dealing with obstacles. Some high schools, for example, allow new mothers special time to breastfeed.

Breastfeeding advice and public acceptance seem a long way from research. But these outside factors can have very real effects on the science. If fact, the researchers have to account for the extent of their teenage subjects' breastfeeding knowledge. That's why Kertz, a lactation consultant, met with the girls in their study from delivery onward, to provide breastfeeding basics.

Still, the researchers at the Houston center don't know exactly how the teens handled their breastfeeding before their study began. Theresa O. Scholl, who is with the University of Medicine and Dentistry of New Jersey, read Motil's paper on breast milk production. Scholl's career has focused on the effects of teen pregnancy and lactation on the health of girls and their infants.

> ✎ **Weird Words**
>
> Lactation: The process of a mother's body making milk for an infant.
>
> Nursing: Breastfeeding.

"The differences between the growing teens and adult women in this study are huge. It's really impressive," says Scholl. "It might be good to do a follow-up study of the infants from birth to the first 6 months. That way, you could find out if the teen mothers were offering to nurse less often from the start and if that contributed to a reduction in milk flow."

Kertz agrees that the study's findings, like all scientific research, open the door to new questions.

"Breastfeeding is an issue of supply and demand," she says. "The more a mother breastfeeds, the more milk she'll have and the longer she'll be able to nurse. Most of the girls weaned their infants at 3 to 4 months. Was this an arbitrary decision to stop nursing, or did the young mothers lack the nutrients to continue?"

♣ **It's A Fact!!**

Recent studies suggest that teens' growth continues during pregnancy.

There are bigger questions, however—the most basic one being how real is the competition between growing teens and their infants for nutrients? Another is: Do the girls really continue to grow during their childbearing and nursing? Medical textbooks once said no; now the question is being revisited.

Scholl points to her studies of pregnant teens that measured growth of the lower leg only, rather than from head to foot. Lordosis, a natural bending of the spine during pregnancy, can cause errors in a head-to-foot measurement. These studies suggested strongly that growth continues during pregnancy.

Does it follow that continued growth in teens could affect breast milk volume? Scholl points out that, during pregnancy at least, nature often favors the mother during nutrient stress. Studies on famine and infant birth weight have suggested this natural advantage may have contributed to the survival of the human species.

"Nature wouldn't allow the mother to deplete all her resources," says Scholl. "If it did, she couldn't live to bear more offspring. Moreover, if the mother died, what would happen to her baby?"

More research will need to be done to say with certainty that teen growth causes nutrient competition that results in lower birth weights in newborns and less milk during lactation. But Scholl's work on teen births and Motil's work on teen nursing lend support to the theory that the body puts some of its nutrients on reserve to benefit the teenage mother.

If this proves to be true, physicians will want to be sure that teenage mothers are getting the extra nutrition they and their infants need to ensure breastfeeding success.

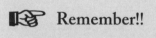 **Remember!!**

Teenage mothers may need extra nutrition to ensure breastfeeding success.

Chapter 14

Food Label Makes Good Eating Easier

Tortilla chips. Chocolate pudding. Frozen yogurt. Allison Gilliam, 16, of Gaithersburg, Maryland, points out some of her favorite foods at her neighborhood grocery store.

Sliced turkey. Dried fruit. The list of items goes on. They're all delicious, and you might never guess that they're also all low in or without fat. Even the chocolate pudding!

It says so right on the food label, and Gilliam, a high-school junior, spots the information right away. A front-label fat claim draws her to the product, and she finds the Nutrition Facts panel on the side or back of the package with more complete information.

Gilliam uses the food label to help her control her fat intake. "I used to be fat," she says. "I lost 45 pounds."

She knows dietary fat is the most concentrated source of calories (9 calories per gram versus 4 calories per gram for carbohydrate and protein), so she checks the label to see how much fat a food contains. If the fat content is over 5 grams per serving, she considers buying something else instead.

About This Chapter: The text in this chapter is from "On the Teen Scene: Food Label Makes Good Eating Easier" by Paula Kurtzweil, Publication No. (FDA) 98-2294. The article originally appeared in the September 1995 *FDA Consumer*; this version contains revisions made in December 1997.

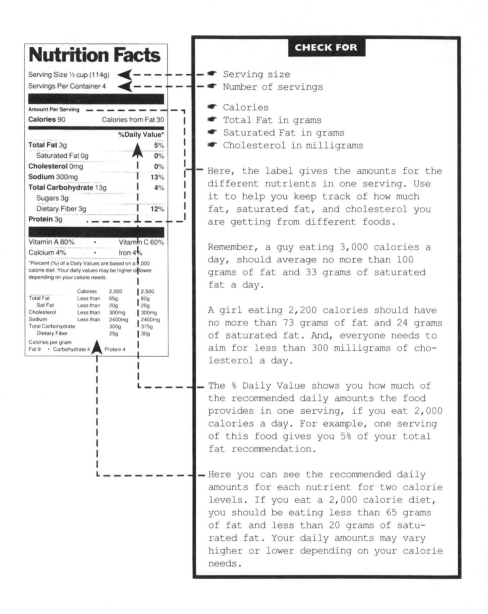

Nutrition Facts

Serving Size ½ cup (114g)
Servings Per Container 4

CHECK FOR

☞ Serving size
☞ Number of servings

Amount Per Serving

Calories 90   Calories from Fat 30

☞ Calories
☞ Total Fat in grams
☞ Saturated Fat in grams
☞ Cholesterol in milligrams

%Daily Value*

Total Fat 3g	5%
Saturated Fat 0g	0%
Cholesterol 0mg	0%
Sodium 300mg	13%
Total Carbohydrate 13g	4%
Sugars 3g	
Dietary Fiber 3g	12%
Protein 3g	

Vitamin A 80%   •   Vitamin C 60%

Calcium 4%   •   Iron 4%

*Percent (%) of a Daily Values are based on a 2,000 calorie diet. Your daily values may be higher or lower depending on your calorie needs.

		Calories	2,000	2,500
Total Fat		Less than	65g	80g
Sat Fat		Less than	20g	25g
Cholesterol		Less than	300mg	300mg
Sodium		Less than	2400mg	2400mg
Total Carbohydrate			300g	375g
Dietary Fiber			25g	30g

Calories per gram
Fat 9   •   Carbohydrate 4   •   Protein 4

Here, the label gives the amounts for the different nutrients in one serving. Use it to help you keep track of how much fat, saturated fat, and cholesterol you are getting from different foods.

Remember, a guy eating 3,000 calories a day, should average no more than 100 grams of fat and 33 grams of saturated fat a day.

A girl eating 2,200 calories should have no more than 73 grams of fat and 24 grams of saturated fat. And, everyone needs to aim for less than 300 milligrams of cholesterol a day.

The % Daily Value shows you how much of the recommended daily amounts the food provides in one serving, if you eat 2,000 calories a day. For example, one serving of this food gives you 5% of your total fat recommendation.

Here you can see the recommended daily amounts for each nutrient for two calorie levels. If you eat a 2,000 calorie diet, you should be eating less than 65 grams of fat and less than 20 grams of saturated fat. Your daily amounts may vary higher or lower depending on your calorie needs.

Figure 14.1. Understanding Nutrition Facts labels. (Source: Hearty Habits: Don't Eat Your Heart Out," National Heart, Lung, and Blood Institute, Pub. No. 93-3102, September 1993.)

Like Gilliam, you can make the food label work for you—whether your concern is losing weight, gaining weight, eating enough protein, eating less fat, or simply staying in the good shape you're in.

New Label

The food label was revamped in 1994, thanks to regulations from the Food and Drug Administration and the U.S. Department of Agriculture. As a result, you get:

- easy-to-read nutrition information required on almost every packaged food

- %Daily Values, which show how a serving of food fits into a total day's diet

- serving sizes that are closer to the amounts most people actually eat than previous labeling

- nutrition claims that mean the same on every product

> ♣ **It's A Fact!!**
>
> Dietary fat is the most concentrated source of calories—9 calories per gram versus 4 calories per gram for carbohydrate and protein.

- voluntary information for the most commonly eaten fresh fruits and vegetables, and raw fish and cuts of meat. This information may appear on posters or in brochures in the same area as the food.

Get The Facts

The main draw is the "Nutrition Facts" panel, which gives information about nutrients people are most concerned about today. For example, the panel gives the lowdown on fat, saturated fat, and cholesterol because of their link to heart disease.

You may find particularly useful information about nutrients that teenagers especially need. For instance, girls, who often eat fewer calories than boys, sometimes don't get enough calcium and iron, so they can use the label to help them choose foods that give a good supply of those nutrients. Girls also have special needs for these nutrients: Consumption of milk and other products containing calcium in teen years may help prevent osteoporosis later in life; extra iron is sometimes needed to replace what's lost during menstruation.

Almost everyone wants to know about calorie content. For sports-minded teens, getting enough calories may be the concern, while those who tend to be overweight may want to reduce their calorie intake. The food label can help because it almost always will list the calories in a serving of food.

✎ Weird Words

When these words appear on food labels, they have specific meanings.

Fat-Free: Less than 0.5 g fat per serving.

Good Source Of Calcium: At least 100 milligrams (mg) calcium per serving.

High-Protein: At least 10 grams (g) high-quality protein per serving.

Light (two meanings):

- One-third fewer calories or half the fat of the reference food. (If 50 percent or more of the food's calories are from fat, the fat must be reduced by 50 percent.)
- A "low-calorie," "low-fat" food whose sodium content has been reduced by 50 percent of the reference food

Low-Fat: 3 g or less fat per serving. (If the serving size is 30 g or less or 2 tablespoons or less, 3 g or less fat per 50 g of the food.)

More Iron: At least 1.8 mg more iron per serving than reference food. (Label will say 10 percent more of the Daily Value for iron.)

Reduced Or Fewer Calories: At least 25 percent fewer calories per serving than the reference food.

Sugar-Free: Less than 0.5 g sugar per serving.

%Daily Values

The amount of nutrients in a food is given in one or two ways: in grams (or milligrams) or as a percentage of the Daily Value, a new label reference tool.

The %Daily Value shows how a serving of food fits in with current recommendations for a healthful daily diet. These reference numbers—called Daily Values—are based on the government's Dietary Guidelines; for example, one guideline recommends restricting fat intake to 30 percent or less of calorie intake.

The government has set 2,000 calories a day as the basis for calculating %Daily Values. Of course, not everyone eats this amount. Teenage girls often average 2,200 calories a day, while some teen-age boys may eat 2,500 or more calories a day.

Whatever your calorie intake, you still can use the %Daily Values on the label to get a general idea of how a serving of food fits into the total daily diet.

The goal is to eat about 100 percent of the Daily Value for each nutrient each day. For nutrients that may be related to health problems—such as fat, saturated fat, and sodium—100 percent should be the upper limit. For other nutrients that are often needed to maintain good health and which may be in short supply—such as fiber and calcium—the goal is to eat at least 100 percent.

A good rule of thumb: If the %Daily Value listed on the panel is 5 or less, the food contributes a small amount of that nutrient to the diet.

Nutrient Claims

Just as Gilliam does for low-fat products, you can easily spot foods offering the kind of nutritional benefits you want by looking for claims on the package.

The government has set strict definitions for 12 "core" terms:

• free	• light	• high
• reduced	• extra lean	• more
• lean	• low	• good source
• less	• fewer	• healthy

These terms can be used only if the food meets certain criteria, so when you see them, you can believe them.

Health Claims

Another type of claim, the health claim, also can alert you to nutritious foods. FDA has approved 10 claims. They show a link between:

- calcium and a lower risk of osteoporosis. The claim must state that regular exercise and a healthy diet with enough calcium helps teen and young adult white and Asian women maintain good bone health and may reduce their high risk of osteoporosis later in life.

- fat and a greater risk of cancer

- saturated fat and cholesterol and a greater risk of heart disease

- fiber-containing grain products, fruits and vegetables and a reduced risk of cancer

- fruits, vegetables and grain products that contain fiber and a reduced risk of heart disease

- sodium and a greater risk of high blood pressure

- fruits and vegetables and a reduced risk of cancer

- folic acid and a decreased risk of neural tube defects in fetuses. Neural tube malformations are serious birth defects that cause disability or death.

- dietary sugar alcohols and a reduced risk of cavities

- soluble fiber from whole oats, as part of a diet low in saturated fat and cholesterol, and a reduced risk of heart disease.

Look For The Info

The food label won't tell you what foods to eat—that's your decision—but it will help you find foods with the kinds of nutritional benefits you want.

Also, many fast-food places voluntarily offer nutrition information about their foods. The information is often available on request. Many of these restaurants now offer low-fat choices, including lettuce salads and low-fat entrees.

So, like teenage Gilliam, you, too, may soon find yourself eating a whole new way. In Gilliam's case, that's a low-fat diet that includes such foods as baked tortilla chips, fat-free pudding, nonfat frozen yogurt, and skim milk. After all, said Gilliam, "It's second nature to me now."

☞ Remember!!

Food labels won't tell you what foods to eat—that's your decision—but they will help you find foods with the kinds of nutritional benefits you want.

Chapter 15

Assessing School Lunches

The National School Lunch Program (NSLP) is one of the best-known Federal Government programs. During fiscal 1995, about 26 million children in just over 94,000 schools and residential childcare institutions participated in the program, at a Federal cost of about $5.1 billion—up about 3 percent since fiscal 1994.

The NSLP provides lunches to children in public and nonprofit private schools and residential child-care institutions. The U.S. Department of Agriculture (USDA) provides schools with cash and commodities to partially offset the cost of the program's food and foodservice. Additional cash is provided to subsidize lunches for low-income children. To participate in the program, schools must serve lunches that meet Federal nutritional requirements and offer free and reduced-price lunches to children determined eligible for such benefits.

A recent study sponsored by USDA showed that, averaged over one week, school lunches in the NSLP provided nutritious food to the Nation's school children at reasonable prices. However, on average, lunches are high in fat, saturated fat, and sodium, and some fall short of the Recommended Dietary Allowance (RDA) for key nutrients for some age groups.

About This Chapter: The text in this chapter is from "Public and Private Efforts for the National School Lunch Program" by Charlene Price and Betsey Kuhn in *Food Review*, May-August 1996 v18 n2 p51(7). *Food Review* is a publication of the U.S. Department of Agriculture.

The regulations surrounding the NSLP were amended in 1995 in response to evolving knowledge about nutrition and the dietary needs of Americans. NSLP lunch menus are required to meet critical nutritional needs by the 1996-97 school year. Waivers may be granted by individual State agencies for up to 2 years to allow schools time to train foodservice employees and to accommodate other special circumstances.

Through the "School Meals Initiative for Healthy Children," USDA is working with school foodservice personnel to provide nutritious and palatable meals with less fat and sodium and more fiber. Through the program, efforts are also underway to educate school foodservice workers and children about nutrition. Schools are also experimenting with allowing private firms to enter the school lunch market. Such public-private partnerships have led to the development of more nutritious fast food products for use in school lunch menus.

Goals Evolved Along With Nutrition Knowledge

The dietary goals of the NSLP have been based on food guidance information made available by USDA. This nutrition information has evolved over time to incorporate the latest information about the relationship of diet to health.

The National School Lunch Act of 1946 established the NSLP to "safeguard the health and well-being of our Nation's children." Nutritional concerns at that time centered around reducing nutrient deficiencies due to underconsumption of food. In particular, at the time, military recruits were failing physical fitness requirements thought to be caused, in part, by nutrient deficiencies. The Act sought to address underconsumption by requiring NSLP meals to provide balanced nutrition and minimum amounts of specific food groups—meat/meat alternate, bread/bread alternate, vegetables/fruits, and milk—amounts sufficient to provide one-third of the RDA's for key nutrients.

As nutrient deficiencies due to underconsumption lessened for many children, other nutritional concerns arose. By the 1970's, concerns focused on excessive consumption of fat in many diets. In 1980, the first edition of the

Dietary Guidelines for Americans was published, providing Federal dietary recommendations for healthy Americans ages 2 years and over. These guidelines provided directional changes, focusing attention on the importance of modifying diets to reduce consumption of fat and other components. The *Dietary Guidelines* are reviewed by a panel of experts every 5 years to determine whether the existing recommendations need to be updated based on current scientific findings in the fields of nutrition and health.

In *Dietary Guidelines for Americans*, people are urged to eat a variety of foods; maintain or improve their weight; choose a diet with plenty of grain products, vegetables, and fruits; and choose a diet moderate in sugars, salt, and sodium. The guidelines also recommend that people choose a diet that provides no more than 30 percent of total calories from fat and reducing saturated fat to less than 10 percent of calories.

Focus On Improving The Nutritional Quality Of Meals

Children's diets need improvement to meet the recommendations of the *Dietary Guidelines*. Recent studies show children's overall diets meet the RDA's for most vitamins and minerals, but their intake of total fat, saturated fat, and sodium exceed dietary guideline recommendations. Research has shown that foods prepared away from home are typically higher in fat and saturated fat than are foods prepared at home. School lunches have been no exception.

A 1993 USDA dietary assessment of school meals showed that, on average, school lunches provided foods sufficient to meet approximately one-third or more of the RDA for key nutrients, including vitamins A, C, and B6, and calcium, iron, and zinc. However, school lunches exceeded the recommended levels for fat and saturated fat (average program lunches contained 38 percent of calories from total fat and 15 percent of calories from saturated fat).

In USDA's revision of the nutritional requirements of NSLP meals in 1995, lunches, averaged over a 1-week period, are required to provide one-third of the RDA for protein, vitamins A and C, iron, calcium, and calories. Averaged over a week, lunches must contain no more than 30 percent of calories from fat and less than 10 percent of calories from saturated fat. Schools must conform to these criteria by the 1996-97 school year, unless they received a waiver.

USDA Provides Flexibility To Meet Nutritional Standards

The new regulations provide school foodservice directors with several menu planning options to help them meet the revised nutrition requirements. Under one option, called Nutrient Standard Menu Planning or NuMenus, schools conduct a nutrient analysis on foods offered in the program over a school week. This analysis is done using computer software. Appropriate adjustments are then made to ensure that the meals averaged over the week meet the nutrition standards for key nutrients. When using NuMenus, the traditional five-item-minimum menu requirement (one meat/meat alternate, one bread/bread alternate, two vegetables/fruits, and one milk) would no longer be used. Instead, lunches would have to include a minimum of three menu items—an entree or main course, fluid milk, and one other food item—and meet required nutrition standards.

A second option, called Assisted NuMenus, allows schools to arrange for menu development and nutrition analysis by outside entities, such as State agencies, consortiums of school food authorities, or private consultants.

Schools may opt to continue using the food-based meal pattern for school lunches or they may elect to use another option, which is an enhanced food-based system of menu planning and preparation with increased quantities of

---

✎ Weird Words

Commodities: In the context of this chapter, agricultural products; commodities frequently provided to schools for lunch programs include: fresh, canned, and frozen fruits and vegetables; meats; fruit juices; vegetable shortening; peanut products; vegetable oil; and flour and other grain products.

National School Lunch Program: A federally assisted meal program providing nutritionally balanced, low-cost or free, lunches to eligible school children. Other federal programs include the Special Milk Program and the School Breakfast Program.

vegetables, fruits, and bread/grain products, that meet required nutritional standards over a school week.

There may be other reasonable approaches to meal planning that would achieve compliance with the new NSLP nutrition standards. Therefore, USDA is developing guidelines and a proposed rule that would set criteria for State agencies to use when they consider and approve such approaches.

Improving The Nutritional Quality Of Food Products

In addition to focusing on bettering the meals, USDA is also improving the nutritional quality of the commodities it provides to schools. About 17 percent (1 billion pounds) of the food served in school meals is provided by USDA. The rest is purchased by the schools or by private organizations under contract with the schools. Foods provided by USDA will be:

- *Lower in fat.* For example, the maximum fat content of frozen ground beef and frozen ground pork will be reduced by at least 1 percentage point a year, from 17-19 percent in 1995-96 to 15-17 percent by 1997-98; "light" mozzarella cheese products with maximum fat content of 10.8 percent will be substituted as an alternative to part-skimmed mozzarella, which is up to 21 percent fat; the maximum fat content of reduced-fat peanut butter products will be cut to 12 grams of fat per 2-tablespoon serving.

- *Lower in sodium.* For example, refried beans and canned carrots will have lower salt levels; and the maximum amount of salt in canned tuna and salmon will be reduced from 1.5 percent to about 1 percent.

- *Lower in sugar.* For example, sweet potatoes will be packed in fruit juice instead of syrup; and red tart cherries will also contain reduced sugar levels.

These and other product modifications should contribute significantly toward improving the nutritional content of school lunches.

Improving Food Choices

The meals and food products are not the only targets of USDA's reinvention efforts for the program. School meals also need to be palatable to children

❖ It's A Fact!!

Providing healthy meals is the first important step in improving children's diets. But no meal, however healthy, will have an effect on health unless it is eaten. Team Nutrition is USDA's nationwide program, developed to help schools implement the School Meals Initiative for Healthy Children. The nutrition promotion arm of Team Nutrition is a multifaceted, national effort to provide nutrition education through schools, families, the community, and the media. In addition, Team Nutrition provides training and technical assistance to support foodservice personnel in implementing the *Dietary Guidelines for Americans* in school meals. Team Nutrition will also monitor the implementation and evaluate the success of the program.

Team Nutrition created a network of public-private partnerships to help spread its research-based messages. The Walt Disney Company created two 30-second Team Nutrition Public Service Announcements (PSA's) featuring characters from The Lion King movie. The PSA's are being broadcast regularly on the Disney cable television channel and are available at no cost to all broadcast television stations and cable television services. Supporting posters featuring the Disney characters were also produced for use in schools and communities.

The in-school component of the program has been developed in cooperation with Scholastic, Inc. Together, Team Nutrition and Scholastic have created a nutrition education program that can be integrated into the basic school curriculum. Through this partnership, Team Nutrition expects to reach over 23 million young people and 1.4 million teachers in 90 percent of America's schools.

In cooperation with USDA's Center for Nutrition Policy and Promotion and USDA's Cooperative State Research, Education, and Extension Service, Team Nutrition has developed the Team Nutrition Community Action Kit, which it has distributed through State and local cooperative extension service agencies and to 4-H clubs and the Internet.

Taken together, all these promotion and training activities provide a comprehensive, reinforcing strategy for improving school meals and children's diets.

For more information, visit the Team Nutrition web site at http://fns1.usda.gov/tn.

Source: "USDA Acts To Improve School Meals and Children's Nutrition," *Food Review*, May-August 1996.

participating in the program, so there is minimal food waste. Team Nutrition was created to be the implementation tool for USDA's "School Meals Initiative for Healthy Children." Team Nutrition's two components are technical assistance/training and nutrition education. Its mission is to improve the health and nutrition of children by creating innovative public and private partnerships that promote food choices for a healthy diet. Some existing partnerships include organizations such as The Walt Disney Company, Scholastic Inc., and the National PTA.

Under the technical assistance/training component of Team Nutrition, USDA will provide the education, motivation, and training to school foodservice personnel to provide healthy meals that appeal to children and that meet the *Dietary Guidelines*.

Foodservice Companies Also In On The Act

Faced with dwindling budgets and increased per child lunch costs due to decreased participation in the NSLP, more school foodservice directors are using alternative programs. Approximately 1,000 of the 15,000 school districts in the United States have contracted with foodservice companies to manage their school foodservice programs. Contract foodservice companies have been involved in the school food programs for nearly 50 years. These companies provide complete food management services—offering menu ideas, recipes, employee training, purchasing assistance, inventory control, and other management services.

In 1995, all 330 public schools in Rhode Island contracted with private foodservice companies to manage their school foodservice programs. Since then, local officials report that participation increased and students threw away less food. For example, these schools served 2,652 lunches a day during the 1991-92 school year. In 1995, in schools where private firms provided the cafeteria food, the number of lunches served grew 31 percent. Inspections at several of those elementary schools found that most of the hot-food trays were "completely cleared of food" by the end of the lunch period. The privately managed lunch program for 1 Rhode Island School District, composed of 41 schools, generated a $350,000-savings in the 1994-95 school year through increased revenues and lower costs.

The Salem-Keizer School District in Salem, Oregon, has used private contractors for the lunch programs at its 52 schools for about 15 years. According to local officials, the program spent about $100,000 more than originally budgeted during the last year of the district-run lunch program. Since privatization, the program has saved between $150,000 and $350,000 a year for the district.

Other school districts also report successfully working with private contractors to reduce operating costs of lunch programs, while increasing participation and the nutritional quality of lunches. For example, the five schools in the South Pasadena Unified School District in California reduced costs by about $50,000 a year in food and product costs over the 1993-94 and 1994-95 school years when their lunch program was managed by Marriott, a private foodservice company (the year before Marriott got involved, the lunch program was $30,000 over budget). In addition, fat and sodium levels have been lowered to improve the healthfulness of meals. Lunch participation has increased and plate waste has been decreased by setting up buffet tables where students serve themselves.

The General Accounting Office completed a study in July 1996 of national plate waste in the NSLP. The amount of food thrown away varied by type of food, according to school cafeteria managers. For example, the average amount of waste for cooked vegetables was 42 percent, compared with 11 percent for milk. Almost 80 percent of cafeteria managers believed that allowing students to select only what they want to eat would reduce plate waste.

The major companies providing foodservice to U.S. public schools are Marriott Management Services; Aramark, Inc.; and Daka, Inc.

Marriott, the largest foodservice contractor in the United States, has been in the school foodservice business for 25 years. It operates in 3,500 schools and 350 school districts. Grand Marketplace, one of their secondary-school programs, replicates a food court at school, by offering a choice of eight entrees. This program is designed to facilitate faster service and maximize the use of the facilities. At least once a week a food bar is offered—potato, pizza, bagel, taco, soup, salad, hot dog/hamburger, pasta, chili, and sandwich—where students can build their own meals.

Aramark, the second-largest U.S. foodservice contractor, has catered to schools for 45 years. They have seen a marked increase in their school accounts in the last 5 to 7 years. Aramark is currently in 330 school districts (2,300 schools) across the country.

Massachusetts-based Daka, Inc., has been in school foodservice since 1976. Daka is currently in 60 school districts (100 schools) nationwide. Daka, Inc., is the 10th ranked contract foodservice chain in the United States.

These and other contract foodservice companies are working with USDA and local schools to implement the new regulations for healthful school meals. For example, Marriott is testing a new menu called Healthy School Meals in 12 school districts. It includes 30 recipes modified to be lower in fat.

✤ It's A Fact!!

Profile of USDA's National School Lunch Program, based on fiscal year 1997

- Schools and residential childcare institutions participating: 94,000
- Lunches served daily: 27 million
- Free lunch requirement: Family income below 130 percent of the Federal poverty level ($20,865 for a family of four).
- Reduced-price lunch requirement: Family income from 130 percent to 185 percent of the Federal poverty level ($29,693 for a family of four).

Most of the support USDA provides to schools in the National School Lunch Program comes in the form of a cash reimbursement for each meal served. The current case reimbursement rates are:

- Free meals: $1.89
- Reduced-price meals: $1.49
- Pain meals: 18 cents

Source: U.S. Department of Agriculture's Food and Nutrition Service (FNS), Nutrition Program Facts: National School Lunch Program, December 1997.

> ### ♣ It's A Fact!!
>
> School lunches are required to provide one-third of the RDA for protein, vitamins A and C, iron, calcium, and calories, while school breakfasts must provide one-fourth of the day's allowance for those nutrients and calories. Both lunches and breakfasts averaged over a 1-week period must contain no more than 30 percent of calories from fat and less than 10 percent of calories from saturated fat.

These companies also offer a wide variety of educational materials focusing on nutrition education tailored for students in kindergarten through grade 12. These range from interactive classroom lesson plans and videos on exercise and nutrition; to songs, games, quizzes, and cards filled with fun facts, to computer nutrition education programs that stress the importance of eating a variety of foods by acquainting students with the Food Guide Pyramid.

Fast Food Chains Adding To The Menu

Fast food chains are recent entrants into school foodservice. They are a small but growing component of those providing meals for the program. In schools, fast food chains offer limited food fare. Fast food items offered as part of a NSLP meal must meet USDA nutrition requirements, requiring some items to be modified. (Fast food fare is also offered in some schools "a la carte," with each food item offered and priced separately from NSLP meals. These a la carte items are priced higher than the same product is priced when included in the NSLP meal. Students receiving a NSLP school meal can buy extra food a la carte, but they pay full price for the food.)

The number of schools serving fast food is low but growing. Currently, approximately nine fast food chains sell to schools across the country: Pizza Hut, Little Caesar's, Domino's, Taco Bell, Subway, Chick-fil-A, McDonald's, Blimpie's, and Arby's. (Little Caesar's, Domino's, and McDonald's are not aggressively pursuing the school lunch market and are not monitoring the number of schools they serve. Arby's and Blimpie's are in fewer than 50 schools.)

PepsiCo's Pizza Hut has the highest school presence, in approximately 5,000 of the just over 94,000 schools across the country in 1994-95, up from

4,000 in 1992-93. Pizza Hut offers several one-topping pizzas to schools—pepperoni pizza and cheese pizza are the most popular among the students. Two other pizza chains offer similar products in the school lunch market nationwide—Domino's and Little Caesar's. Under the nutrient-based option, the pizza does not have to be modified. But under the food-based option, the pizza would have to be modified to meet the 2-ounce protein requirement set up by the NSLP.

Schools are increasingly offering "brand days," in which the school rotates the fast food chains' products with regular cafeteria offerings. Several school districts report that lunch participation increases on the days that brand name, fast food products are sold. For example, Capital Hill Schools in Dover, Delaware, added Pizza Hut products at high schools in 1994 when seniors were allowed to go off-campus for lunch. NSLP meal participation in those high schools rose 18 percent on the days Pizza Hut products were sold. Brand day rotations also lessen on-site labor requirements because the food arrives at the school fully prepared.

McDonald's was the first chain to offer products in school lunch programs—approximately 20 years ago. McDonald's currently offers two products to schools—hamburgers and cheeseburgers. In some schools, students cannot buy the burger a la carte. They must buy the complete school lunch as part of the NSLP, which also includes school-prepared french fries, salad, and milk.

Taco Bell, another subsidiary of PepsiCo, Inc., is the largest U.S. chain serving Mexican food. Taco Bell entered school foodservice in 1992 and served around 2,000 schools nationwide in 1994-95. Their catering programs provide schools with a fresh prepared product delivered directly to the school cafeteria. Taco Bell's catered products include a bean burrito, beef burrito, combination bean and beef burrito, and a chili cheese burrito. In order to meet USDA's nutrient requirement for protein, additional beans, meat, or cheese are added to their regular retail products for service at schools.

Another approximately 350 schools are licensed to prepare and serve Taco Bell tacos and burritos. The school purchases food supplies from the chain, and the chain trains the school staff to prepare the product. A line of frozen Taco Bell food products is also served in those schools.

Taco Bell is the only chain that has designed a lower fat menu especially for schools, although two of its four specially designed products exceed the limit of 30 percent of calories from fat as outlined in the *Dietary Guidelines*: chicken bean enchiladas have 35 percent of their calories from fat, and fiesta casseroles have 34 percent of calories from fat. Taco Bell's chicken burritos have 30 percent of calories from fat, and 27 percent of calories in Taco Bell's Border pizza are from fat.

Subway has served sandwiches in approximately 1,000 schools nation-wide since 1992. These are delivered cold and without mayonnaise. Subway's cold-cut sandwiches are less than 30 percent of calories from fat. Their products do not have to be modified in any way and are sold in most schools under a licensing or catered program. Subway sandwiches can be included in the NSLP meal plan or can be sold a la carte.

Chick-fil-A, Inc., has been in schools since 1992. The chain delivers a fried chicken-fillet sandwich, with 27 percent of calories from fat, to schools for their lunch program. Chick-fil-A currently services about 500 schools and the number is growing.

Arby's is new to the school lunch circuit. The chain started a pilot program with the San Juan Unified School District in California in early 1995. Prewrapped roast beef sandwiches are delivered hot daily in special insulated containers to 10 of the district's 19 secondary schools. Sandwiches are modified to contain 2-ounce portions of beef (with a sauce package) to qualify as part of a NSLP lunch. The school district plans to expand the program to all 19 of their secondary schools by the end of the 1996-97 school year.

In 1995, Blimpie International entered into a partnership with public school foodservices in one district in Colorado and two on Long Island, New York. They set up a quick-service counter in schools to sell the company's standard menu, but the school foodservice staff operates the unit.

Blimpie's cold cut sandwiches are offered under the NSLP and also sold a la carte. Under the NSLP, however, sandwiches are modified to meet the protein requirements.

On Tomorrow's Menu

Parents and school and government officials have expressed concern about the nutritional value of the fast food products in school lunches—with some being over the 30 percent of calories from fat allowance. However, the chains insist that under the new regulations, fast food products can be incorporated into week-long menus that average the fat content to acceptable levels.

The Government and private vendors are working together to bring more tasty, nutritious, healthy meals to our Nation's school children. USDA is working with contract foodservice companies to help them comply with new regulations. Already, Marriott, Aramark, and Daka are testing new, healthier products and menus in some school districts to see which ones the students like.

Manufacturers and processors have developed many new lowfat and low-sodium products—such as light butter, lowfat macaroni and cheese, prune puree (as a fat substitute), meatless spaghetti sauce, and boneless turkey ham—that can be useful in meeting the NSLP requirements.

In addition to changing the foods and meals, USDA has joined with private companies and public groups to provide nutrition information for children and their parents to promote life-long healthy food choices.

☞ Remember!!

The National School Lunch Program (NSLP) provides lunches to children in public and nonprofit private schools and residential child-care institutions. To participate in the program, schools must serve lunches that meet Federal nutritional requirements and offer free and reduced-price lunches to children determined eligible for such benefits.

In 1995 the U.S. Department of Agriculture (USDA) revised the nutritional requirements of NSLP meals. Averaged over a 1-week period, meals are required to provide one-third of the RDA for protein, vitamins A and C, iron, calcium, and calories. Averaged over a week, lunches must contain no more than 30 percent of calories from fat and less than 10 percent of calories from saturated fat.

But no meal, however healthy, will have an effect on health unless it is eaten.

Chapter 16

Eating Well While Eating Out

Between school, your part-time job, and band practice, you barely have time to scarf down a piece of pizza with some soda. You've heard the drill from your health teacher about the importance of eating well, but how are you supposed to do that when your schedule is so demanding and you're hardly ever at home? Read this chapter to find out how busy teens can eat well while eating out.

The Importance Of Eating Well

A slice of pizza every once in a while won't do you any harm, but you should be careful to eat a healthy diet.

Stephanie Smith, MS, RD, spokesperson for the Colorado Dietetic Association, puts it in perspective. "If you take care of your 'insides,' you'll notice a difference in your 'outsides.' Hair, teeth, and skin are just a few of the 'outsides' that reflect what we eat . . . so are strength, energy, and concentration."

Eating at fast-food restaurants or the mall may not sound like a very healthy choice. Even dining in the school cafeteria can be a problem. But it's easy to make good choices in these kinds of situations. All you have to do is plan ahead. Smith tells teens that this is critical, because one third of their total calories are usually consumed away from home.

If I Eat Well At Home, What's Wrong With Splurging When I Eat Out?

Occasionally eating less-than-healthy foods isn't a big problem, but frequent splurging may be an obstacle to good health.

The U.S. Food and Drug Administration (FDA) developed the Food Guide Pyramid to help us make healthy food choices. It's easy to use because it recommends what to eat but is not a rigid prescription. Using the Food Guide Pyramid to make food choices helps ensure that you eat a variety of foods to maximize nutrients and the right amount of food to maintain a healthy weight.

> ♣ **It's A Fact!!**
>
> The food you eat affects your:
>
> • mental functioning
> • emotional well-being
> • energy
> • strength
> • weight
> • future health

According to the FDA, average food intake over a few days—not a single meal—is what's important. If you eat a meal consisting of junk food, for example, try to balance it with healthier foods the rest of that day and the next.

The good news is this means you don't have to eat perfectly all the time. It's OK to splurge every once in a while, as long as your diet is generally good.

Eating On The Go

Eating healthy on the run doesn't have to be hard.

To maximize your nutrient intake for the day, start each day with breakfast. "It increases metabolism and energy, allowing your brain to function more effectively," says Jessica Donze, RD, CDN, a pediatric nutrition therapist in Wilmington, Delaware. "That means better school performance, better athletic performance, and more calories burned."

And wherever you are eating, Donze recommends fitting in fruits and vegetables whenever possible. "Preferences and habits can be learned," Donze says. "You need 5 servings (combined) of fruits and vegetables each day. The truth is, you can't eat too many vegetables. This change will help your body get the vitamins and fiber it needs."

Isn't it harder to eat healthy foods away from home? Actually, it just takes some practice. Here are some healthy suggestions for teens who are on the run or away from home.

At A Restaurant

The Center for Science in the Public Interest (CSPI), an organization dedicated to improving the safety and nutritional quality of our food, suggests requesting the following foods and types of preparation when eating in restaurants:

- Sauces and salad dressings should be served on the side and used sparingly. Use low-calorie dressings.
- Ask for half-portions (or take home half).
- Use of salsa and mustard instead of mayonnaise or oil.
- Ask for olive or canola oil instead of butter, margarine, or shortening.
- Nonfat or low-fat milk should be used instead of whole milk or cream.
- Order baked, broiled, or grilled (not fried) lean meats including turkey, chicken, seafood, or sirloin steak.
- Salad, vegetables, or baked potatoes make healthier side dishes than french fries. Use a small amount of sour cream instead of butter on a baked potato.
- Treat yourself to fresh fruit instead of sugary, high-fat desserts.

At The Mall

It's tempting to pig out while shopping, but with a little planning, it's easy to eat healthy foods at the mall. Smith recommends these choices:

- single slice of veggie pizza
- small hamburger
- bean burrito
- baked potato

> **✔ Quick Tip**
>
> Increasing the amount of fruits and vegetables in your daily diet will help you eat a more nutritionally balanced diet whether you are eating at home or out. Nutritionists recommend five servings from the fruit and vegetable food group per day.

- side salad
- frozen yogurt
- grilled, not fried, sandwiches (for example, a grilled chicken breast sandwich)

Resist the temptation to "super size" your meals. This can add up to 25% more fat and calories. The American Dietetic Association also recommends that when you have a craving for something unhealthy, try sharing it with a friend.

In The School Cafeteria

The suggestions for eating in a restaurant and at the mall apply in the high-school or university cafeteria as well. Add vegetables and fruit whenever possible, and opt for the leaner, lighter items. Go easy on the high-fat, low-nutrition items, such as mayonnaise, fried foods, and heavy salad dressings.

You might want to consider packing your own lunch occasionally. Here are some lunch items that pack a healthy punch:

- Sandwiches with lean meats or fish, like turkey, chicken, tuna (made with low-fat mayo), lean ham, or lean roast beef. For variety, try other sources of protein, like peanut butter, hummus, or meatless chili.

- Low-fat or nonfat milk, yogurt, or cheese

- Any fruit that's in season

- Raw baby carrots, green and red pepper strips, tomatoes, or vegetable juice

- Whole-grain breads, pita, bagels, or crackers

☞ Remember!!

It can be easy to achieve a healthy diet, even on the run. If you develop the skills to make healthy choices now, your body will thank you later.

Chapter 17

Soft Drinks And Your Health

In 1942, when production of carbonated soft drinks was about 60 12-ounce servings per person, the American Medical Association's (AMA) Council on Foods and Nutrition stated:

> From the health point of view it is desirable especially to have restriction of such use of sugar as is represented by consumption of sweetened carbonated beverages and forms of candy which are of low nutritional value. The Council believes it would be in the interest of the public health for all practical means to be taken to limit consumption of sugar in any form in which it fails to be combined with significant proportions of other foods of high nutritive quality.[1]

By 1998, soft-drink production had increased by nine-fold and provided more than one-third of all refined sugars in the diet, but the AMA and other medical organizations now are largely silent. This review discusses the nutritional impact and health consequences of massive consumption of soft-drinks,[2] particularly in teenagers.

✎ Weird Words

Ascorbic Acid: Vitamin C; important in forming collagen, a protein that gives structure to bones, cartilage, muscle, and blood vessels. It also helps to maintain capillaries, bones, and teeth and aids in the absorption of iron.

Caffeine: A mildly addictive stimulant drug, present in coffee and most cola and "pepper" drinks, as well as in some orange sodas and other products.

Calcium: A mineral used for building bones and teeth and in maintaining bone strength; also used in muscle contraction, blood clotting, and maintenance of cell membranes.

Carbonated: Added carbon dioxide to make bubbly or fizzy.

Dental Caries: cavities in the teeth; tooth decay.

Insulin Resistance: A condition in which the body does not respond properly to the action of insulin, a hormone that helps the body use glucose (sugar) for energy.

Kidney Stones: In the kidney, a collection of minerals that are part of a person's normal diet; developed from crystals that separate from urine and build up on the inner surfaces of the kidney.

Magnesium: a mineral used in building bones, manufacturing proteins, releasing energy from muscle storage, and regulating body temperature.

Obesity: A condition of having 20 percent (or more) extra body fat for age, height, sex, and bone structure.

Osteoporosis: A disease in which bone mass is reduced and the risk of fractures is increased.

Riboflavin: Vitamin B$_2$; a water-soluble vitamin, helps the body release energy from protein, fat, and carbohydrates during metabolism.

Sugar: A class of carbohydrates that taste sweet; types are lactose, glucose, fructose, and sucrose.

Vitamin A: A fat-soluble vitamin involved in the formation and maintenance of healthy skin, hair, and mucous membranes; also helps us to see in dim light and is necessary for proper bone growth, tooth development, and reproduction.

Soaring Consumption Of Soft Drinks

Carbonated soft drinks account for more than 27 percent of Americans' beverage consumption.[3] In 1997, Americans spent over $54 billion to buy 14 billion gallons of soft drinks. That is equivalent to more than 576 12-ounce servings per year or 1.6 12-ounce cans per day for every man, woman, and child.[4] That is also more than twice the amount produced in 1974. Artificially sweetened diet sodas account for 24% of sales, up from 8.6% in 1970.[5]

Children start drinking soda pop at a remarkably young age, and consumption increases through young adulthood. One fifth of one- and two-year-old children consume soft drinks.[6] Those toddlers drink an average of seven ounces—nearly one cup—per day. Toddlers' consumption changed little between the late 1970s and mid 1990s.

Almost half of all children between 6 and 11 drink soda pop, with the average drinker consuming 15 ounces per day. That's up slightly from 12 ounces in 1977-78.

The most avid consumers of all are 12- to 29-year-old males. Among boys 12 to 19, those who imbibe soda pop drink an average of almost 2½

Table 17.1. Consumption of non-diet soft drinks by 12- to 19-year-olds (ounces per day) and percent of caloric intakes (all figures include non-drinkers).

Year	Ounces per day		Percent of calories	
	boys	girls	boys	girls
1977-78	7	6	3	4
1987-88	12	7	6	5
1994-96	19	12	9	8

Source: Calculated from U.S. Dept. Agr. Nationwide Food Consumption Survey, 1977-78; Continuing Survey of Food Intakes by Individual, 1987-88, 1994-96.

12-ounce sodas (28.5 ounces) per day. Teenage girls also drink large amounts of pop. Girls who drink soft drinks consume about 1.7 sodas per day. (Women in their twenties average slightly more: two 12-ounce sodas per day.) (See Tables 17.1 and 17.2)

In a new analysis of diet-intake data, soft-drink consumption by 13- to 18-year-olds was examined (the results cannot be compared directly to the data shown for 12- to 19-year-olds because slightly different methods were used). This analysis identified how much soda pop is consumed by how many teens. For instance, one-fourth of 13- to 18-year-old male pop-drinkers drink 2½ or more cans per day, and one out of 20 drinks five cans or more.[7] (See Table 17.3) One-fourth of 13- to 18-year-old female pop-drinkers drink about two cans or more per day, and one out of twenty drinks three cans or more.[8] (Actual intakes may well be higher, because many survey participants tend to underestimate quantities of "bad" foods consumed.)

By contrast, twenty years ago, the typical (50th-percentile) 13- to 18-year-old consumer of soft drinks (boys and girls together) drank ¾ of a can per day, while the 95th-percentile teen drank 2¼ cans. That's slightly more than one-half of current consumption.

Table 17.2. Consumption of regular and diet soft drinks by 12- to 19-year-olds (excludes non-drinkers).

Year	Ounces per day	
	boys	girls
1977-78	16	15
1987-88	23	18
1994-96	28	21

Source: U.S. Dept. Agr. Nationwide Food Consumption Survey, 1977-78; Continuing Survey of Food Intakes by Individual, 1987-88, 1994-96.

Table 17.3. Consumption of regular and diet soft drinks by 13- to 18-year olds (ounces per day; excludes non-drinkers)

	percentiles					
	5	25	50	75	90	95
1994-96 boys, 13-18	6	12	20	30	44	57
1994-96 girls, 13-18	4	6	14	23	32	40
1977-78 boys and girls	3	5	9	15	-	27

Source: Percentile calculations by Environ, Inc.; data from USDA, CSFII, Figures for 1977-78 calculated from P.M. Guenther, *J. Am. Diet. Assoc.* 1986;86:493-9.

One reason, aside from the ubiquitous advertising, for increasing consumption is that the industry has steadily increased container sizes. In the 1950s, Coca-Cola's 6½-ounce bottle was the standard serving. That grew into the 12-ounce can, and now those are being supplanted by 20-ounce bottles (and the 64-ounce Double Gulp at 7-Eleven stores). The larger the container, the more beverage people are likely to drink, especially when they assume they are buying single-serving containers.

Also, prices encourage people to drink large servings. For instance, at McDonald's restaurants a 12-ounce ("child size") drink costs 89 cents, while a drink 250% larger (42-ounce "super size") costs only 79% more ($1.59).[9] At Cineplex Odeon theaters, a 20-ounce ("small") drink costs $2.50, but one 120% larger (44-ounce "large") costs only 30% more ($3.25).[10]

Nutritional Impact Of Soft Drinks

Regular soft drinks provide youths and young adults with hefty amounts of sugar and calories. Both regular and diet sodas affect Americans' intake of various minerals, vitamins, and additives.

Sugar Intake

Carbonated drinks are the single biggest source of refined sugars in the American diet.[11] According to dietary surveys,[12] soda pop provides the average American with seven teaspoons of sugar per day, out of a total of 20 teaspoons. Teenage boys get 44% of their 34 teaspoons of sugar a day from soft drinks. Teenage girls get 40% of their 24 teaspoons of sugar from soft drinks. Because some people drink little soda pop, the percentage of sugar provided by pop is higher among actual drinkers.

The U.S. Department of Agriculture (USDA) recommends that people eating 1,600 calories a day not eat more than six teaspoons a day of refined sugar, 12 teaspoons for those eating 2,200 calories, and 18 teaspoons for those eating 2,800 calories.[13,14] To put those numbers in perspective, consider that the average 12- to 19-year-old boy consumes about 2,750 calories and 1½ cans of soda with 15 teaspoons of sugar a day; the average girl consumes about 1,850 calories and one can with ten teaspoons of sugar. Thus, teens just about hit their recommended sugar limits from soft drinks alone. With candy, cookies, cake, ice cream, and other sugary foods, most exceed those recommendations by a large margin.

> ♣ **It's A Fact!!**
>
> • Boys aged 12 to 19 who drink soda pop drink an average of 28 ounces per day.
>
> • Girls aged 12 to 19 who drink soda pop drink an average of 21 ounces per day.
>
> • One out of four 13- to 18-year-old male soda pop-drinkers drink 2½ or more cans per day, and one out of 20 drinks five cans or more.
>
> • One out of four 13- to 18-year-old female soda pop-drinkers drink about two cans or more per day, and one out of twenty drinks three cans or more.

Calorie Intake

Lots of soda pop means lots of sugar means lots of calories. Soft drinks are the fifth largest source of calories for adults.[15] They provide 5.6% of all the calories that Americans consume.[16] In 12- to 19-year-olds, soft drinks provide 9% of boys' calories and 8% of girls' calories.[17] Those percentages are triple (boys) or double (girls) what they were in 1977-78. (See Table 17.1) Those figures include teens who consumed little or no soda pop.

For the average 13- to 18-year-old boy or girl drinker, soft drinks provide about 9% of calories. Boys and girls in the 75th percentile of consumption obtained 12% of their calories from soft drinks, and those in the 90th percentile about 18% of their calories.

Nutrient Intakes

Many nutritionists state that soft drinks and other calorie-rich, nutrient-poor foods can fit into a good diet. In theory, they are correct, but, regrettably, they ignore the fact that most Americans consume great quantities of soft drinks and meager quantities of healthful foods. One government study found that only 2% of 2- to 19-year-olds met all five federal recommendations for a healthy diet.[18] USDA's Healthy Eating Index found that on a scale of 0-100, teenagers had scores in the low 60s (as did most other age-sex groups). Scores between 51 and 80 indicate that a diet "needs improvement."[19]

Dietary surveys of teenagers found that in 1996:

- Only 34% of boys and 33% of girls consumed the number of servings of vegetables recommended by USDA's Food Pyramid.

- Only 11% of boys and 16% of girls consumed the recommended amount of fruit.

- Only 29% of boys and 10% of girls consumed the recommended amount of dairy foods.

- Most boys and girls did not meet the recommended amounts of grain and protein foods.

Those surveys also found that few 12- to 19-year-olds consumed recommended amounts of certain nutrients, including:

- *calcium*: only 36% of boys and 14% of girls consumed 100% of the Recommended Dietary Allowance (RDA).

- *vitamin A*: only 36% of boys and 31% of girls consumed 100% of the RDA.

- *magnesium*: only 34% of boys and 18% of girls consumed 100% of the RDA.

As teens have doubled or tripled their consumption of soft drinks, they cut their consumption of milk by more than 40%. Twenty years ago, boys consumed more than twice as much milk as soft drinks, and girls consumed 50% more milk than soft drinks. By 1994-96, both boys and girls consumed twice as much soda pop as milk (and 20- to 29-year-olds consumed three times as much). Teenage boys consumed about 2 2/3 cups of carbonated soft drinks per day but only 1¼ cups of fluid milk. Girls consumed about 1½ cups per day of soft drinks, but less than 1 cup of milk. Compared to adolescent nonconsumers, heavy drinkers of soda pop (26 ounces per day or more) are almost four times more likely to drink less than one glass of milk a day.[20]

In 1977-78, teenage boys and girls who frequently drank soft drinks consumed about 20% less calcium than non-consumers. Heavy soft-drink consumption also correlated with low intake of magnesium, ascorbic acid, riboflavin, and vitamin A, as well as high intake of calories, fat, and carbohydrate.[21] In 1994-96, calcium continued to be a special problem for female soft-drink consumers.[22]

Health Impact Of Soft Drinks

The soft-drink industry has consistently portrayed its products as being positively healthful, saying they are 90% water and contain sugars found in nature. A poster that the National Soft Drink Association has provided to teachers states:

> As refreshing sources of needed liquids and energy, soft drinks represent a positive addition to a well-balanced diet....These same three sugars also occur naturally, for example, in fruits....In your body it makes no difference whether the sugar is from a soft drink or a peach.[23]

M. Douglas Ivester, Coca-Cola's chairman and CEO, defending marketing in Africa, said, "Actually, our product is quite healthy. Fluid replenishment is a key to health....Coca-Cola does a great service because it encourages people to take in more and more liquids."[24]

In fact, soft drinks pose health risks both because of what they contain (for example, sugar and various additives) and what they replace in the diet (beverages and foods that provide vitamins, minerals, and other nutrients).

Obesity

Obesity increases the risk of diabetes and cardiovascular disease and causes severe social and psychological problems in millions of Americans. Between 1971-74 and 1988-94, obesity rates in teenage boys soared from 5% to 12% and in teenage girls from 7% to 11%. Among adults, between 1976-80 and 1988-94, the rate of obesity jumped by one-third, from 25% to 35%.[25]

Numerous factors—from lack of exercise to eating too many calories to genetics—contribute to obesity. Soda pop adds unnecessary, non-nutritious calories to the diet, though it has not been possible to prove that it (or any other individual food) is responsible for the excess calories that lead to obesity. However, one recent study found that soft drinks provide more calories to overweight youths than to other youths. The difference was most striking among teenage boys: Soda pop provides 10.3% of the calories consumed by overweight boys, but only 7.6% of calories consumed by other boys. There was no consistent pattern of differences with regard to intake of calories, fat, or several other factors.[26]

Obesity rates have risen in tandem with soft-drink consumption, and heavy consumers of soda pop have higher calorie intakes.[27] While those observations do not prove that sugary soft drinks cause obesity (heavy consumers may exercise more and need more calories), heavy consumption is likely to contribute to weight gain in many consumers.

Regardless of whether soda pop (or sugar) contributes to weight gain, nutritionists and weight-loss experts routinely advise overweight individuals to consume fewer calories—starting with empty-calorie foods such as soft drinks. The National Institutes of Health recommends that people who are trying to lose or control their weight should drink water instead of soft drinks with sugar.[28]

Bones And Osteoporosis

People who drink soft drinks instead of milk or other dairy products likely will have lower calcium intakes. Low calcium intake contributes to osteoporosis, a disease leading to fragile and broken bones.[29] Currently, 10 million Americans have osteoporosis. Another 18 million have low bone mass and are at increased

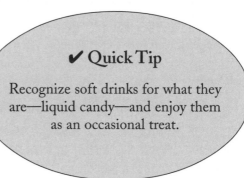

✔ **Quick Tip**

Recognize soft drinks for what they are—liquid candy—and enjoy them as an occasional treat.

risk of osteoporosis. Women are more frequently affected than men. Considering the low calcium intake of today's teenage girls, osteoporosis rates may well rise.

The risk of osteoporosis depends in part on how much bone mass is built early in life. Girls build 92% of their bone mass by age 18,[30] but if they don't consume enough calcium in their teenage years they cannot "catch up" later. That is why experts recommend higher calcium intakes for youths 9 to 18 than for adults 19 to 50. Currently, teenage girls are consuming only 60% of the recommended amount, with soft-drink drinkers consuming almost one-fifth less than nonconsumers.[31]

While osteoporosis takes decades to develop, preliminary research suggests that drinking soda pop instead of milk can contribute to broken bones in children. One study found that children 3 to 15 years old who had suffered broken bones had lower bone density, which can result from low calcium intake.[32]

Tooth Decay

Refined sugar is one of several important factors that promote tooth decay (dental caries). Regular soft drinks promote decay because they bathe

the teeth of frequent consumers in sugar-water for long periods of time during the day. An analysis of data from 1971-74 found a strong correlation between the frequency of between-meal consumption of soda pop and dental caries.[33] (Those researchers considered other sugary foods in the diet and other variables.) Soft drinks appear to cause decay in certain surfaces of certain teeth more than in others.[34]

Tooth-decay rates have declined considerably in recent decades, thanks to such preventive factors as fluoride-containing toothpaste, fluoridated water, tooth sealants, and others. Nevertheless, caries remains a problem for some people. A large survey in California found that children (ages 6 to 8, 15) of less-educated parents have 20% higher rates of decayed and filled teeth.[35] A national study found that African-American and Mexican-American children (6 to 18 years old) are about twice as likely to have untreated caries as their white counterparts.[36] For people in high-risk groups, prevention is particularly important.

To prevent tooth decay, even the Canadian Soft Drink Association recommends limiting between-meal snacking of sugary and starchy foods, avoiding prolonged sugar levels in the mouth, and eating sugary foods and beverages with meals. Unfortunately, many heavy drinkers of soft drinks violate each of those precepts.

Heart Disease

Heart disease is the nation's number-one killer. Some of the most important causes are diets high in saturated and trans fat and cholesterol; cigarette smoking; and a sedentary lifestyle. In addition, in many adults a diet high in sugar may also promote heart disease.

High-sugar diets may contribute to heart disease in people who are "insulin resistant." Those people, an estimated one-fourth of adults, frequently have high levels of triglycerides and low levels of HDL ("good") cholesterol in their blood. When they eat a diet high in carbohydrates, their triglyceride and insulin levels rise. Sugar has a greater effect than other carbohydrates.[37] The high triglyceride levels are associated with a higher risk of heart disease.[38] It would make sense for insulin-resistant people, in particular, to consume low levels of regular soft drinks and other sugary foods. Research is needed on insulin resistance in adolescents.

Kidney Stones

Kidney (urinary) stones are one of the most painful disorders to afflict humans and one of the most common disorders of the urinary tract. According to the National Institute of Diabetes and Digestive and Kidney Diseases (NIDDK), a unit of the National Institutes of Health, more than 1 million cases of kidney stones were diagnosed in 1985.[39] NIDDK estimates that 10 percent of all Americans will have a kidney stone during their lifetime. Several times more men, frequently between the ages of 20 and 40, are affected than women. Young men are also the heaviest consumers of soft drinks.

After a study suggested a link between soft drinks and kidney stones, researchers conducted an intervention trial.[40] That trial involved 1,009 men who had suffered kidney stones and drank at least 5 1/3 ounces of soda pop per day. Half the men were asked to refrain from drinking pop, while the others were not asked. Over the next three years drinkers of Coca-Cola and other cola beverages acidified only with phosphoric acid who reduced their consumption (to less than half their customary levels) were almost one-third less likely to experience recurrence of stones. Among those who usually drank soft drinks acidified with citric acid (with or without phosphoric acid), drinking less had no effect. While more research needs to be done on the cola-stone connection, the NIDDK includes cola beverages on a list of foods that doctors may advise patients to avoid.

Additives

Several additives in soft drinks raise health concerns. Caffeine, a mildly addictive stimulant drug, is present in most cola and "pepper" drinks, as well as some orange sodas and other products. Caffeine's addictiveness may be one reason why six of the seven most popular soft drinks contain caffeine.[41] Caffeine-free colas are available, but account for only about 5% of colas made by Coca-Cola and Pepsi-Cola.[42] On the other hand, Coca-Cola and other companies have begun marketing soft drinks, such as Surge, Josta, and Jolt, with 30% to 60% more caffeine than Coke and Pepsi.

In 1994-96, the average 13- to 18-year-old boy who drank soft drinks consumed about 1 2/3 cans per day. Those drinking Mountain Dew would have ingested 92 mg of caffeine from that source (55 mg caffeine/12 ounces).

That is equivalent to about one six-ounce cup of brewed coffee. Boys in the 90th-percentile of soft-drink consumption consume as much caffeine as is in two cups of coffee; for girls the figure is 1½ cups of coffee.

One problem with caffeine is that it increases the excretion of calcium in urine.[43] Drinking 12 ounces of caffeine-containing soft drink causes the loss of about 20 milligrams of calcium, or two percent of the U.S. RDA (or Daily Value). That loss, compounded by the relatively low calcium intake in girls who are heavy consumers of soda pop, may increase the risk of osteoporosis.

Caffeine can cause nervousness, irritability, sleeplessness, and rapid heart beat.[44] Caffeine causes children who normally do not consume much caffeine to be restless and fidgety, develop headaches, and have difficulty going to sleep.[45] Also, caffeine's addictiveness may keep people hooked on soft drinks (or other caffeine-containing beverages). One reflection of the drug's addictiveness is that when children age six to 12 stop consuming caffeine, they suffer withdrawal symptoms that impair their attention span and performance.[46]

Several additives used in soft drinks cause occasional allergic reactions. Yellow 5 dye can cause asthma, hives, and a runny nose.[47] A natural red coloring, cochineal (and its close relative carmine), can cause life-threatening reactions.[48] Dyes can cause hyperactivity in sensitive children.[49]

In diet sodas, artificial sweeteners may raise concerns. Saccharin, which has been replaced by aspartame in all but a few brands, has been linked in human studies to urinary-bladder cancer and in animal studies to cancers of the bladder and other organs.[50] Congress has required products made with saccharin to bear a warning label. The safety of acesulfame-K, which was approved in 1998 for use in soft drinks, has been questioned by several cancer experts.[51]

Aggressive Marketing Of Soft Drinks

Soft-drink companies are among the most aggressive marketers in the world. They have used advertising and many other techniques to increase sales.

Soft-drink advertising budgets dwarf all advertising and public-service campaigns promoting the consumption of fruits, vegetables, healthful diets, and low-fat milk. In 1997, Coca-Cola, which accounts for 44%[52] of the soft-drink market in the U.S., spent $277 million on advertising and the four major companies $631 million. Between 1986 and 1997 those companies spent $6.8 billion on advertising.[53]

Companies make sure their products are always readily accessible. Thus, in 1997, 2.8 million soft-drink vending machines dispensed 27 billion drinks worth $17.5 billion.54 Coca-Cola's soft drinks are sold at two million stores, more than 450,000 restaurants, and 1.4 million vending machines and coolers.[55]

The major companies target children aggressively (though, to their credit, they have not gone after 4-year-olds by advertising on Saturday-morning television). Pepsi advertises on Channel One, a daily news program shown in 12,000 schools.[56] Companies inculcate brand loyalties in children and boost consumption by paying school districts and others for exclusive marketing

Table 17.4. Beverage prices.

Beverage	Cost	Cost per quart (¢)
Cola, supermarket brand	$.59/2 liters	28
Coca-Cola	$.69/2 liters	33
Pepsi-Cola	$.99/6 12-oz. cans; $3.99/24 12-oz. cans	44
Bottled water, (supermarket brand)	$.79/gallon	20
Bottled spring water, (supermarket brand)	$.89/gallon	22
Seltzer water, club soda, supermarket brand	$.89/2 liters	42
Milk	$2.79/gallon; $.95/quart	70; 95
Orange juice, frozen, supermarket brand	$1.39/12-oz. can	93

Source: Prices at Washington-area supermarkets, September, 1998.

agreements. For instance, Dr Pepper paid the Grapevine-Colleyville, Texas, School District $3.45 million for a ten-year contract (it includes rooftop advertising to reach passengers in planes landing at the nearby Dallas/Ft. Worth Airport).[57] To reach youths after school, Coca-Cola is paying $60 million over ten years to the Boys & Girls Clubs of America for exclusive marketing rights in more than 2,000 clubs.[58]

Pepsi, Dr Pepper, and Seven-Up encourage feeding soft drinks to babies by licensing their logos to a major maker of baby bottles, Munchkin Bottling, Inc. Infants and toddlers are four times likelier to be fed soda pop out of those bottles than out of regular baby bottles.[59]

Also fueling soft-drink sales is the low cost of the sugar-water-additive products. (See Table 17.4) Supermarket brands are particularly cheap, easily getting as low as 28 cents per quart, but even Coca-Cola and Pepsi-Cola are available for 33 cents per quart when on special. Milk costs two to three times as much, about 70 to 95 cents per quart.

Moreover, in recent years, inflation has had a greater effect on the price of milk than of soft drinks. Between 1982-84 and 1997 the Consumer Price Index rose 2.3 times as much for milk as for soft drinks.[60]

The soft-drink industry is aiming for continued expansion in coming years. Thus, the president of Coca-Cola bemoans the fact that his company accounts for only 1 billion out of the 47 billion servings of all beverages that earthlings consume daily.[61] The company's goal is to:

> make Coca-Cola the preferred drink for any occasion, whether it's a simple family supper or a formal state dinner. . . . [T]o build pervasiveness of our products, we're putting ice-cold Coca-Cola classic and our other brands within reach, wherever you look: at the supermarket, the video store, the soccer field, the gas station—everywhere.[62]

Recommendations For Action [from the Center for Science in the Public Interest]

In part because of powerful advertising, universal availability, and low price, and in part because of disinterest on the part of many nutritionists and other health professionals, Americans have come to consider soft drinks a routine snack and a standard, appropriate part of meals instead of an occasional treat, as they were treated several decades ago. Moreover, many of today's younger parents grew up with soft drinks, see their routine consumption as normal, and so make little effort to restrict their children's consumption of them.

It is a fact, though, that soft drinks provide enormous amounts of sugar and calories to a nation that does not meet national dietary goals and that is experiencing an epidemic of obesity. The replacement of milk by soft drinks in teenage girls' diets portends continuing high rates of osteoporosis. Soft drinks may also contribute to dental problems, kidney stones, and heart disease. Additives may cause insomnia, behavioral problems, and allergic reactions and may increase slightly the risk of cancer.

☞ Remember!!

Many nutritionists state that soft drinks and other calorie-rich, nutrient-poor foods can fit into a good diet. In theory, they are correct, but, regrettably, they ignore the fact that most Americans consume great quantities of soft drinks and meager quantities of healthful foods.

Soft drinks pose health risks both because of what they contain (for example, sugar and various additives) and what they replace in the diet (beverages and foods that provide vitamins, minerals, and other nutrients).

- Carbonated drinks are the single biggest source of refined sugars in the American diet.

- Soft drinks provide 5.6% of all the calories that Americans consume.

- As teens have doubled or tripled their consumption of soft drinks, they cut their consumption of milk by more than 40%.

Teens should consider how much soda pop they are drinking, and if appropriate, make dietary changes.

The industry promises that it will be doing everything possible to persuade even more Americans to drink even more soda pop even more often. Parents and health officials need to recognize soft drinks for what they are—liquid candy—and do everything possible to return those beverages to their former, reasonable role as an occasional treat.

- Individuals and families should consider how much soda pop they are drinking and reduce consumption accordingly. Parents should stock their homes with healthful foods and beverages that family members enjoy.

- Physicians, nurses, and nutritionists routinely should ask their patients how much soda pop they are drinking and advise them, if appropriate, of dietary changes to make.

- Organizations concerned about women's and children's health, dental and bone health, and heart disease should collaborate on campaigns to reduce soft-drink consumption.

- Local, state, and federal governments should be as aggressive in providing water fountains in public buildings and spaces as the industry is in placing vending machines everywhere.

- State and local governments should considering taxing soft drinks, as Arkansas, Tennessee, Washington, and West Virginia already do. Arkansas raised $40 million in fiscal year 1998 from that tax.[63] If all states taxed soft drinks at Arkansas' rate (2 cents per 12-ounce can), they could raise $3 billion annually. Those revenues could fund campaigns to improve diets, build exercise facilities (bike paths, swimming pools, etc.), and support physical-education programs in schools.

- Local governments could require calorie listings on menu boards at fast-food outlets and on vending machines to sensitize consumers to the nutritional "cost" of sugared soft drinks and other foods.

- School systems and other organizations catering to children should stop selling soft drinks, candy, and similar foods in hallways, shops, and cafeterias.

- School systems and youth organizations should not auction themselves off to the highest bidder for exclusive soft-drink marketing rights. Those deals profit the companies and schools at the expense of the students' health.

- The National Academy of Sciences or Surgeon General should review the impact of current and projected levels of soft-drink (and sugar) consumption on public health.

- Soft-drink companies voluntarily should not advertise to children and adolescents. Labels should advise parents that soft drinks may replace lowfat milk, fruit juice, and other healthy foods in the diets of children and adolescents.

- Scientific research should explore the role of heavy consumption of soft drinks (and sugar) in nutritional status, obesity, caries, kidney stones, osteoporosis, and heart disease.

Notes

1. *JAMA*. 1942;120:763-5.

2. This review does not cover sweetened non-carbonated beverages (bottled ice teas, fruit drinks and ades, bottled ice tea, etc.).

3. National Soft Drink Assoc. web site, http://www.nsda.org/.

4. Ibid.

5. USDA/ERS: Food Consumption, Prices, and Expenditures, 1970-95, *Stat. Bull. No. 939* (August, 1997).

6. Unless otherwise specified, all data on consumption of soft drinks, milk, and calorie intake were obtained or calculated from U.S. Department of Agriculture (USDA) surveys (one-day data) particularly Continuing Survey of Food Intakes of Individuals (CSFII), 1994-96 (Data Tables 9.4, 9.7, 10.4, 10.7); 1987-88 (Report No. 87+1, Tables 1.2-1 and -2; 1.7-1 and -2); Nationwide Food Consumption Surveys, 1977-78 (Tables A1.2-1 and -2; A1.7-1and -2). Intake of added sugars by age was obtained from USDA's analysis for purposes of the Food Guide Pyramid (two-day 1996 data, Table 6). Teens' consumption of vegetables, fruit, and other foods also is from Pyramid Servings Data, USDA, Dec. 1997, based on CSFII, 1996. We are grateful to USDA staff members in the

Food Surveys Research Group for their assistance. (See USDA web site: www.barc.usda.gov/bhnrc/foodsurvey/home.htm)

7. Analyses by Environ, Inc., Sept. 1998, based on USDA CSFII 1994-96 two-day data.

8. Ibid.

9. CSPI survey, August 26, 1998.

10. *Nutrition Action Healthletter*. 1998 (July/Aug.);25(6):6.

11. *Am. J. Clin. Nutr*. 1995;62(suppl):178S-94S.

12. Those dietary surveys find that consumers report consuming only 57% of all soft drinks produced. While some soft drinks are wasted or returned to manufacturers, that fact provides good evidence that the surveys greatly underestimate actual intake.

13. U.S. Dept. Agr. The Food Guide Pyramid. *Home and Garden Bulletin No. 252*, Oct. 1996, p. 17.

14. USDA's recommendation applies to diets that include 30% of calories from fat. Because 33% of the calories teens consume come from fat, there is even less room in the diet for added sugar.

15. *J. Am. Diet Assoc*. 1998;98:537-547.

16. USDA CSFII 1994-96.

17. Diet sodas, which provide no calories, constitute only 4% of soft-drink consumption by teenage boys and 11% by teenage girls.

18. *Pediatrics*. 1997;100:323-9. *Pediatrics*. 1998;101:952-3.

19. USDA, Center for Nutrition Policy and Promotion, CNPP-5; The Healthy Eating Index, 1994-96, July 1998.

20. Personal communication, Lisa Harnack, Sept. 22, 1998.

21. *J. Am. Diet. Assoc*. 1986;86:493-9.

22. Analyses by Environ, Inc., see note 7. Calcium was the only micronutrient examined.

23. National Soft Drink Assoc. "Soft Drinks and Nutrition." Washington, D.C. (undated).

24. *New York Times.* May 26, 1998, p.D1.

25. *Arch. Pediatr. Adolesc. Med.* 1995; 149:1085-91. *Morbidity Mortality Weekly Report.* March 7, 1997;46(9):199-201.

26. Troiano RP, et al. "Energy and fat intake of children and adolescents in the United States. Data from the National Health and Nutrition Examination Surveys." *Am. J. Clin. Nutr.* In press.

27. Analyses by Environ, see note 7.

28. "Embrace Your Health! Lose Weight if You Are Overweight" NHLBI and Office of Research on Minority Health, NIH Publication No. 97-4061, Sept. 1997.

29. National Osteoporosis Foundation. "Fast facts on osteoporosis." Web site, www.nof.org/stats.html.

30. Institute of Medicine. *Dietary Reference Intakes: Calcium, Phosphorus, Magnesium, Vitamin D, and Fluoride.* 1997; pp.4-28.

31. Analyses by Environ, see note 7.

32. *J. Bone Miner. Res.* 1998;13:143-8.

33. *J. Am. Dent. Assoc.* 1984;109:241-5.

34. *J. Am. Dent. Assoc.* 1972;85:81-89.

35. The Dental Health Foundation. "A Neglected Epidemic: The Oral Health of California's Children." (San Rafael, 1997).

36. *J. Am. Dent. Assoc.* 1998;129:1229-1238.

37. *Am. J. Clin. Nutr.* 58(Suppl); 1993:800S. *J. Clin. Endocrin. Metab.* 1984;59:636.

38. *J. Am. Med. Assoc.* 1996;276:882-8.

39. National Institute of Diabetes and Digestive and Kidney Diseases, web site, http://www.niddk.nih.gov/

40. *J. Clin. Epidemiol.* 1992 (Aug);45(8):911-916.

41. *Beverage Digest* web site, www.beverage-digest.com/980212.html.

42. Ibid.

43. *Osteoporosis Intern.* 1995;5:97-102.

44. American Psychiatric Association. *Diagnostic and Statistical Manual of Mental Disorders.* (Washington, D.C.), 4th ed. 1994.

45. *J. Nervous Mental Disease* 1981;169:726. *Arch. Gen. Psychiat.* 1984;41:1073.

46. *J. Am. Acad. Child Adolesc. Psychiatry.* 1998;37:858-65.

47. *Federal Register.* 1979;44:37212-37221.

48. *Ann. Allergy Asthma Immunol.* 1997;79:415-9.

49. *Science.* 1980;207:1487.

50. *Lancet* 1980;i:837-840. *Env. Health Perspectives* 1998;25:173-200.

51. Associated Press. "Consumer group attacks artificial sweetener." Aug. 1, 1996.

52. *Beverage World* web site, http://www.beverageworld.com/.

53. *Beverage Digest* web site (data expressed in 1998 dollars).

54. *Vending Times*, 1998;38(9):15,21,22.

55. *Wall Street Journal*, May 8, 1997, p.1.

56. *Wall Street Journal*, Sept. 15, 1997, B1.

57. *Selling to Kids*, August 19, 1998, p. 4.

58. *Chronicle of Philanthropy.* July 30, 1998, p.25.

59. *ASDC J. Dent. Child.* 1997 (Jan-Feb);64(1):55-60.

60. Bureau of Labor Statistics, U.S. Department of Labor.

61. Coca-Cola Co. Annual Report, 1997; M. Douglas Ivester's introductory statement.

62. Coca-Cola Co. Annual Report, 1997.

63. Arkansas Department of Finance and Administration, Little Rock, Ark.

Chapter 18

Caffeine: Are You Addicted?

"As soon as I wake up in the morning, I head to the refrigerator, and pop open a can of cola. That's my breakfast. Each can gives me 140 calories and a great caffeine lift," said John Grabrick of Little Canada, Minnesota. "I don't like coffee or tea. But I like caffeine's jolt, so I started drinking Coke. Now I go through eight 12-ounce cans each day. This 24-pack will last me three days."

When John was asked how much caffeine he gets every day, he checked the back of a can and started to calculate numbers on a piece of paper. "Hmm, my eight cans add up to 96 ounces a day. I just read that a 12-ounce can contains 46 milligrams (mg) of caffeine. When I divide 46 mg by 12, I get 3.8 mg of caffeine per ounce of cola."

John popped open a can of cold cola and took a long swallow. "To figure out how much caffeine I get, I multiply 96 ounces by 3.8. That comes to 364.8 mg of caffeine every day. Is that a lot?"

Well, one cup of coffee contains about 135 mg of caffeine. John takes in as much caffeine as someone who drinks three cups of coffee a day.

The Inside Scoop

John's caffeine intake is high, but not unusual. Many teens are addicted to caffeine and don't know it—colas, cafe lattes, coffee, espresso, cappuccino,

About This Chapter: The text in this chapter is from "Caffeine's Hook," by Judy Monroe in *Current Health 2*, January 1998 v24 n5 p16(4), © 1998 Weekly Reader Corporation; reprinted with permission.

hot or iced tea, chocolate candy bars, caffeine-laced bottled water and soft drinks are all culprits. If you don't get your daily cola, coffee, tea, or chocolate, do you get headaches?

If you answered "yes," you've got lots of company. Caffeine is the world's most popular drug. On any given day, four of five Americans take it through a variety of drinks, foods, and many prescription and over-the-counter (OTC) or nonprescription drugs such as pain relievers, cold and allergy medicines, diuretics, and diet pills.

More than 60 plant species contain caffeine in their leaves, seeds, or fruits. But the big four plant sources are coffee beans, tea leaves, cocoa pods from

> ✎ **Weird Words**
>
> Caffeine: A stimulant from one of more than 60 plant species, primarily coffee beans, tea leaves, cocoa pods, and kola nuts; odorless and slightly bitter tasting.
>
> Chocolate: A food made from cocoa pods
>
> Coffee: A beverage made from roasted and ground seeds (called beans) of a plant belonging to the *Coffea* genus.
>
> Cola: A carbonated beverage flavored with extract from kola nuts.

which chocolate is made, and kola nuts that are used to flavor colas. Manufacturers add caffeine to other products such as soft drinks, water, and some medications. Because it's a popular flavor, coffee is added to foods such as ice cream, frozen yogurt, candies, cakes, cookies, and muffins. And who can count all the chocolate treats available?

In its pure form, caffeine is odorless and tastes slightly bitter. Although legal and naturally occurring, caffeine is a drug. It's a stimulant. All stimulants excite the central nervous system by increasing the heart rate, breathing, and blood pressure. They also can make people more alert and peppy. But that's not all stimulants do.

Quite A Jolt?

Caffeine, whether consumed in coffee, soft drinks, or in any other form, affects everyone differently. Some people get jittery, nervous, or restless, while others feel energetic. It can change sleep patterns by delaying sleep, or it can cause insomnia, especially if consumed in the evening.

People sometimes become addicted to caffeine, which means they need to take it regularly. Caffeine use creates both dependence and tolerance. An addict is someone who is dependent on a drug and craves its effects. When you drink coffee, tea, or caffeine-laced soft drinks regularly, caffeine dependency can occur within a few days to a couple weeks.

Users can develop a tolerance for caffeine. The body needs more and more of it to feel the same lift. That's what happened to John. He didn't start off drinking so much Coke; but over time, he needed more to keep feeling energetic.

The flip side of dependency is withdrawal. If regular users can no longer get caffeine, withdrawal sets in within 12 to 24 hours. Common caffeine withdrawal symptoms include headaches, anxiety, and fatigue.

John explained how fast caffeine withdrawal can occur. He was scheduled for knee surgery on a Wednesday morning. "The Tuesday before the

---

✔ **Quick Tip**

If you want or need to cut down on caffeine, here are some tips:

- Substitute caffeine-free beverages such as decaffeinated coffee, decaf or herbal teas, and caffeine-free soft drinks.

- Try fruit juices or fruit-flavored all-natural soft drinks. Be wary of fruit-flavored energy drinks that contain caffeine.

- Look for the words caffeine-free on the label of soft drinks and energy drinks, to be certain of what you're getting.

- Choose baked goods, ice cream, and candy that do not contain chocolate or coffee.

- Avoid combination pain relievers, cold remedies, and stay-awake pills.

- If you're not sure whether something contains caffeine, read the product labels and list of ingredients.

Table 18.1. Caffeine Counts

Soft Drinks	Caffeine, milligrams (mg) per 12-ounce can
Jolt™	72
Mountain Dew™	54
Surge™	53
Mellow Yellow™	53
Colas	35-47
Sunkist Orange Soda	41

Hot Drinks	Caffeine (mg)
Starbucks 16 oz "grande"	550
Starbucks coffee, 8 oz "short"	250
Coffee, 8 oz	135
Cappuccino, 8 oz	117
Espresso, 1.5-2 oz cup	100
Cappuccino, 8 oz	61
Cafe latte, 8 oz	61
Cafe mocha, 8 oz	61
Instant coffee, 6 oz	35 to 169
Tea, brewed, 6 oz	25 to 110
Tea, instant, 1 rounded teaspoon for 6 oz cup	31
Hot cocoa, 5 oz	2-20

Treats	Caffeine (mg)
Coffee ice cream, 1 cup	40-60
Coffee yogurt, 1 cup	45
Baking chocolate (used in brownies), unsweetened, 1 oz	26
Dark semisweet chocolate, 1 oz	5-35
Milk chocolate, 1 oz	1-15
Chocolate milk, 1 cup	2-7
Chocolate syrup, 1 oz	4

Prescription Medications	Caffeine (mg)
Cafergot™ (for migraine headaches)	100
Fiorinal™ (for tension headaches)	40
Soma™ (for pain relief, muscle relaxant)	32
Darvon Compound™ (for pain relief, muscle relaxant)	32

OTC Pain Medications	Caffeine (mg)
Excedrin™, 1 tablet	65
Anacin™, 1 tablet	32
Midol™, 1 tablet	32

surgery, I couldn't eat or drink anything after 9 p.m. When I woke up Wednesday morning, I had a huge headache and felt irritable. They wheeled me into surgery and gave me anesthesia to knock me out. When I woke up after the operation with a severe headache, the first words I mumbled to my mom were, 'Get me a Coke.'"

Like caffeine withdrawal, addiction can also occur quickly. Caffeine goes to work fast, within 15 to 45 minutes. Its energy boost does not last long, though. When it wears off, the person feels tired and sluggish, and wants more caffeine to get back its kick.

Limit Use

Experts agree that for most people, a daily soft drink or cup of coffee, with fewer than 240 mg of caffeine, generally causes no harm for adults. However, compared to adults, most teens are smaller in size. So it takes less caffeine a day to reach their limit: a bottle of iced tea, a cup of coffee, or two 12-ounce cans of soft drinks with caffeine.

Heavy daily use—the amount in 4 cups of coffee (about 600 mg)—can result in sleep problems, restlessness, depression, rapid heartbeat, and anxiety. Because it creates more stomach acid, it can cause stomach pains or heartburn. Consuming even higher amounts of caffeine can also give you headaches, muscle pain, shaking, and ringing in the ears.

☞ **Remember!!**

Although caffeine is in our food and drink, it is a drug—one to which many people can become addicted.

Cold and allergy remedies, diet pills, and stimulants that claim to keep people awake all contain caffeine. One to two tablets of an OTC stimulant or diet aid equals one to two cups of coffee in caffeine content. Pain relievers and cold/allergy medicines contain a little less than that amount (see Table 18.1).

Because of health concerns, some people stop consuming caffeine cold turkey: They stop taking anything containing caffeine. Abruptly cutting out caffeine may mean a week of withdrawal symptoms such as fatigue, bad headaches, and drowsiness.

Others slowly cut back on caffeine over two to four weeks. This method reduces or eliminates withdrawal symptoms.

Chapter 19

Food Cravings

Whether you crave a juicy hamburger or a chocolate sundae may depend on whether you're male or female.

A huge mountain of homework looms larger as you get hit with another weekend assignment, your best friend won't speak to you, and now your parents need you to baby-sit your little brother, again. If this chain of events sends you to the kitchen in search of chocolate ice cream or some other sugar- and fat-laden snack, you're not alone.

When stressed, bored, or depressed, it's easy to be overpowered by food cravings. Have you ever found yourself scouring the kitchen for cookies, chips, or even leftover Halloween candy? Then you know how strong cravings can be. And who hasn't heard the stories about pregnant women with bizarre food cravings in the middle of the night?

What causes food cravings has been puzzling scientists for years. Once it was thought they were a signal that your body needed a certain food or nutrient. But research turned up no connection. Some people think it's just a mental thing—it's all in your head. Others believe there's a physical explanation. Although scientists disagree on just what may trigger food cravings, recent research suggests it's a complex combination of physical and mental

About This Chapter: The text in this chapter is from "Food Cravings: Causes and Management," by Sharon Denny in *Current Health 2*, February 1997 v23 n6 p16(3), © 1998 Weekly Reader Corporation; reprinted with permission.

✔ Quick Tip

While the researchers continue to sort out brain chemistry, what do we do about those crazy food cravings? With apologies to David Letterman, here is our "Top 10 List."

1. Manage cravings; don't try to control them. Control often results in failure when you can't ignore that consuming longing for sweets. Manage the craving by satisfying it with one or two cookies or a single scoop of ice cream.

2. Think of cravings as a suggestion to eat, not a demand to overeat. You decide when to eat and how much.

3. Wait it out. Cravings come and go even if you don't feed them. But, give yourself the choice of satisfying it. (See number 1.)

4. Foods are not good or bad. Don't make a list of forbidden foods. It's not the kind of food you eat that adds weight, it's the quantity.

5. Make moderation your goal instead of abstinence.

6. Identify what's causing your craving. Then make a change if you can. For example, your walk home from school takes you by the ice-cream shop. Stopping for one or two scoops is irresistible. Change the route you take or decide to stop only once or twice a week.

7. Eat at least three meals a day. Skipping meals makes you over hungry, which can lead to overeating. Eat a variety of foods to satisfy your hunger. Choose fruits, vegetables, whole grains, low-fat dairy products, and lean meats. Add snacks if you need them.

8. Use creative ways to manage food cravings. For example, all of us have started out to eat just a handful of chips, only to find we've somehow devoured the entire bag. Start with a small bag of chips to manage your munching. Buy single-serving-size packages of cookies, cupcakes, chips, and candy.

9. Get moving. Exercise relieves stress and distracts you from cravings. Walk, skate, dance, swim—whatever gets you moving.

10. Give up guilt, not goodies. One doughnut won't make you fat, but feeling guilty about what you eat might. Feelings of guilt and failure fuel impulsive eating. Enjoying favorite foods occasionally in moderate amounts is an effective way to manage food cravings.

factors. New discoveries in brain chemistry are providing important clues about how food affects our mood.

Males Crave Meat, Females Crave Sweets

Just about everyone experiences food cravings. A survey of college students at McMaster University in Hamilton, Ontario, Canada, found that 97 percent of the women and 68 percent of the men reported an occasional overwhelming desire for certain foods. The number-one pick on the food cravings list of women was chocolate. Women also tended to go for doughnuts, cookies, ice cream, chips, pretzels, and popcorn. For men, it was steak, burgers, fries, and pizza. Although men seem to choose protein foods while women go for carbohydrates, you can see that most foods on both lists are high in fat. Is it possible that we have a "fat tooth" instead of a sweet tooth?

Brain Triggers

Neurotransmitters are chemical messengers sending signals to trigger various feelings and body functions: blood pressure, breathing rate, and appetite, for example. Neurotransmitters include serotonin, which produces feelings of relaxation and calm, and dopamine and norepinephrine, which produce sensations of energy and mental alertness.

Scientists investigating the relationship of food and mood have proposed several theories. But, they don't all agree. Here's a summary of the most popular.

Carbohydrates calm you down. Following an all-carbohydrate snack, levels of the serotonin increase. More serotonin produces feelings of relaxation, but there is a catch. If the carbohydrate food

> ### ✎ Weird Words
>
> Dopamine: A neurotransmitter that is involved in movement.
>
> Neurotransmitters: Chemical messengers sending signals to trigger various feelings and body functions, such as blood pressure, breathing rate, and appetite.
>
> Norepinephrine: A neurotransmitter associated with mood disorders.
>
> Serotonin: A neurotransmitter that affects mood and eating behavior; also important in cycles of waking and sleeping.

also contains fat and/or protein, the effect is lost. Fat slows down digestion, so you don't get the full effect of the carbohydrates.

Protein is another story. Protein does the opposite of carbohydrates: Protein foods perk you up. They contain the amino acid tyrosine that is used to produce dopamine and norepinephrine, the brain chemicals that aid reaction time and mental sharpness. A hunk of meat may not help you ace the math quiz, but it will keep carbohydrates from making you drowsy.

✤ It's A Fact!!

How many doughnuts make a binge? It depends.

Whether a binge is three doughnuts or six depends on your gender. A survey of 400 college students found that eating three doughnuts was described as a binge if the person eating the doughnuts was female. But a guy could eat up to six doughnuts before it was labeled a binge.

According to the researcher, women seem to be more inclined to feel guilty and depressed when they think they have overeaten—which, in turn, could trigger bingeing. Men don't usually express negative emotions; they view eating in more physical terms.

Fat- and sugar-laden foods trigger the brain to release endorphins, chemicals that send out signals of pleasure. Could this explain why the so-called "comfort" foods are mostly high-fat and sweet? The risk here is overeating when anxious or depressed.

So where does chocolate fit in? Chocolate probably boosts endorphins (fat and sugar) and may also raise serotonin levels (carbohydrate). Plus, it contains caffeine, which is a mild stimulant.

🖙 Remember!!

Just about everyone experiences food cravings. Think of cravings as a suggestion to eat, and manage your cravings by satisfying them in moderation. One doughnut won't make you fat, but feeling guilty about what you eat might. Feelings of guilt and failure fuel impulsive eating. Enjoying favorite foods occasionally in moderate amounts is an effective way to manage food cravings.

Chapter 20

Food And Athletic Performance

You've prepared for the game in almost every way possible: you've trained hard with your teammates, heard inspirational speeches from your coach, washed your uniform, and gotten psyched up . . . but now what should you eat?! If this is something you hadn't thought of, you're not alone; many teenage athletes don't really know how to combine food and fitness to reach their potential. And with all the different products available that supposedly make an athlete perform even better, things can get pretty confusing.

The Funky Food Guide Pyramid

Fortunately, eating for sports isn't too complicated or difficult. It actually doesn't even require that you change your diet or buy any special foods or supplements. One of the best ways to ensure you're in top form is to follow the Food Guide Pyramid. Sound simple? It is. By eating the recommended groups of foods in the suggested amounts, you are giving your body the nutrients it needs to succeed. You can find a handy copy of the Food Guide Pyramid on most boxes of cereal. (When following the Food Guide Pyramid, remember that some teenage athletes may need more than the suggested daily servings of certain foods.) Eating regular meals and healthy snacks will keep you in top form.

The Food Guide Pyramid is a crucial part of eating for sports because it includes a huge variety of nutrients. You'll need the combination of vitamins, minerals, protein, carbs, and other nutrients from different foods to be at the top of your game. That's why it's never a good idea to carbohydrate load or eat only one type of food when you're training for an event or game. You may have heard about adults who swear by eating only pasta before a big event, but this isn't the way to go if you're a teenager. A younger body needs different types of foods to do well in sports; eating from only one part of the Food Guide Pyramid will probably let you down.

Eat Extra Calories For Excellence

And while you're picking foods from the Food Guide Pyramid, it's very important that you are eating enough. Dieting is not a part of being an athlete, unless your doctor gives you instructions to do so. Most athletic teenagers need all the calories they normally consume to give them power and strength, and cutting calories can not only hinder performance, it can even be dangerous. In addition, the growth spurts that teenagers undergo require some extra body fat, which translates to extra calories consumed. If anyone—a coach, a gym teacher, or another teammate—says that you should go (or have to go) on a diet, don't do anything until you talk to your doctor. If your doctor determines that a diet is necessary, he or she can work with you to come up with a program that meets your needs. Sometimes your doctor will have you work with a dietitian to get your program going.

> ✎ **Weird Words**
>
> Carbohydrate: One type of nutrient needed by the body; the group includes sugars, starches, and dietary fiber.
>
> Carbohydrate Loading: The practice of manipulating an athlete's diet prior to an endurance competition or event so that it includes a higher than normal amount of carbohydrates.
>
> Dehydration: A condition where the body lacks sufficient fluid.
>
> Food Guide Pyramid: The Food Guide Pyramid is an outline of what to eat each day. It's not a rigid prescription, but a general guide that lets you choose a healthful diet that's right for you. For more information on the Food Guide Pyramid, see Chapter 12.

Supplements, Sports Drinks, And You

Some teenage (and adult) athletes have the idea that while regular food is OK for building strength, supplements and sports foods and drinks must be better for athletes who want to win. Right? The short answer to this idea: wrong. It's easy to get tempted by the hundreds of sports bars, gels, supplements, protein powders, amino acid powders, and other products out there. Their commercials and packages make many promises about building athletes up, increasing their power and strength, and making them healthy, but the real deal is that these products just aren't necessary.

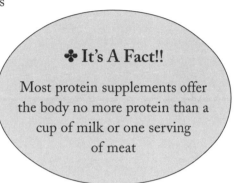

♣ It's A Fact!!

Most protein supplements offer the body no more protein than a cup of milk or one serving of meat

When an athlete drinks a mixture made with a protein product, her body has no idea that it's a sports supplement—it just treats it like plain, regular protein from food. In fact, most protein supplements offer the body no more protein than a cup of milk or one serving of meat, which is usually more tasty, anyway! In other words, these products don't provide you with any more energy that you would get from eating normal food from the Food Guide Pyramid. And normal food is a lot cheaper, too—sports bars and other supplements can deplete your after-school job savings, since they tend to be very expensive.

While none of these supplements do a whole lot of good, they won't really do you too much harm—except in the case of salt tablets. Athletes should never take salt tablets in an effort to compete better. These only serve to dehydrate you and do potential damage to the lining of your stomach—two things that an athlete doesn't need to succeed!

Ditch Dehydration

And speaking of dehydration, don't forget that food isn't the sole key to unlocking your power; water is just as important. When you are perspiring heavily during exercise and your body loses large amounts of water, it's easy to become overheated and not be able to perform to your full potential. In hot or humid weather, heat exhaustion can become a real hazard if you're not staying properly hydrated while you're exercising. The best way to keep hydrated is to drink before, during, and after exercise (or a game or event). The amounts you should drink are as follows:

- 1 to 2 hours before exercising: 10 to 12 ounces of cold water (about 1 1/4 to 1 1/2 cups)

- 10 to 15 minutes before exercising: 10 ounces of cold water (about 1 1/4 cups)

- While exercising: 3 to 4 ounces of cold water every 15 minutes (about a 1/2 cup)

- After exercising: 2 cups of cold water for every pound of weight loss through sweat (this means about a cup or two for most teens; if it's a hot day you may feel thirsty enough to drink even more)

The main thing to remember about staying hydrated is to drink regardless of whether you feel thirsty or not. Thirst is a sign that your body has needed liquids for a while. And when deciding what to grab to quench your thirst, the best drink is cold water—it's the simplest thing for your body to absorb, it's usually easy to find, and it's free! If you like sports drinks, they are

---

✔ Quick Tip

- *Foods to eat 1 to 2 hours before the game or event:* fruit or vegetable juice or fruit (especially plums, melons, cherries, and peaches)

- *Foods to eat 2 to 3 hours before the event:* same as foods above, with bread, a bagel, or an English muffin. (But if you like cream cheese or butter, now is a good time to skip it; the fat in these products could make you feel sick while you're competing.)

- *Foods to eat 3 or more hours before the game or event:* same as foods for 2 to 3 hours before, plus peanut butter, lean meat, low-fat cheese or yogurt, a baked potato, cereal with low-fat milk, or pasta with tomato sauce

also OK, but like sports foods and supplements, they're not necessary for you to get what your body needs. They also tend to be pretty expensive. But if you like the taste and tend to drink more of a sports drink than you would of regular water, then it's fine. If you want to drink water but want a tiny bit of taste, try mixing a splash of juice or a sports drink with the water in a water bottle. But be sure to avoid straight juice or soda, since these contain carbohydrates that could give you a stomachache while you're competing. Also, the caffeine that can be in soda can actually dehydrate you more, which defeats the purpose of drinking in the first place.

Edible Energy

When game day finally rolls around, most of your body's energy will come from the foods you've eaten in the last week, but you can enhance your performance even more by paying attention to the food you eat that day. Foods that are ideal for top performance contain carbohydrates for energy, a small to medium amount of protein, and very little fat.

It's a good practice to avoid eating anything for the hour before you compete, since digestion requires energy—energy that you want to use to win! (Also, eating too soon before certain types of events can cause food to slosh around in your stomach, which can end up leaving you feeling sick and nauseated.) It's also best to avoid candy bars or sodas before your event; these types of foods will give you quick energy, but it won't last long enough.

> **☞ Remember!!**
>
> Eating for sports isn't too complicated or difficult. One of the best ways to ensure you're in top form is to follow the Food Guide Pyramid. By eating the recommended groups of foods in the suggested amounts, you are giving your body the nutrients it needs to succeed.

For more information about healthy eating, check out the Food Guide Pyramid.

Chapter 21

Going Vegetarian

Perceiving plant foods as beneficial because they are high in dietary fiber and, generally, lower in saturated fat than animal foods, many people turn to vegetarian diets.

Grain products, for instance, form the base of the U.S. Department of Agriculture and Department of Health and Human Services' Food Guide Pyramid, which recommends 6 to 11 daily servings of bread, cereal, rice, and pasta. Daily intakes advised for other foods are: 3 to 5 servings of vegetables; 2 to 4 servings of fruits; 2 to 3 servings of milk, yogurt and cheese; and 2 to 3 servings of meat, poultry, fish, dry beans, eggs, and nuts. The guide advises using fats, oils and sweets sparingly.

And, who hasn't seen signs in their grocer's produce section urging consumers to eat "5 a day for better health"? This slogan reflects a major government-industry campaign to help people eat more fruits and vegetables as part of a high-fiber, low-fat diet that emphasizes variety.

The campaign is consistent with the USDA-DHHS Dietary Guidelines for Americans, which states, "Most Americans of all ages eat fewer than the recommended number of servings of grain products, vegetables, and fruits, even though consumption of these foods is associated with a substantially

About This Chapter: The text in this chapter is from "More People Trying Vegetarian Diets" by Dixie Farley, Publication No. (FDA) 96-2296. The article originally appeared in the October 1995 *FDA Consumer*; this version contains revisions made in January 1996.

♣ It's A Fact!!

For people who follow vegetarian diets, the American Dietetic Association has these recommendations:

- Consult a registered dietitian or other qualified nutrition professional, especially during periods of growth, breast-feeding, pregnancy, or recovery from illness.

- Minimize intake of less nutritious foods such as sweets and fatty foods.

- Choose whole or unrefined grain products instead of refined products.

- Choose a variety of nuts, seeds, legumes, fruits, and vegetables, including good sources of vitamin C to improve iron absorption.

- Choose low-fat or nonfat varieties of dairy products, if they are included in the diet.

- Avoid excessive cholesterol intake by limiting eggs, if they are included in the diet, to three or four egg yolks per week.

- For infants, children and teenagers, ensure adequate intakes of calories, vitamin D, calcium, iron, and zinc. (Intakes of vitamin D, calcium, iron, and zinc are usually adequate when a variety of foods and sufficient calories are consumed.)

- If exclusively breast-feeding premature infants or babies beyond 4 to 6 months of age, give vitamin D and iron supplements to the child from birth or at least by 4 to 6 months, as your doctor suggests.

- Usually, take iron and folate (folic acid) supplements during pregnancy.

- In addition, for vegans:

  —Use properly fortified food sources of vitamin B_{12}, such as fortified soy beverages or cereals, or take a supplement.

  —If sunlight is inadequate, take a vitamin D supplement during pregnancy or while breast-feeding.

lower risk for many chronic diseases, including certain types of cancer." Also noted: "Most vegetarians eat milk products and eggs, and as a group, these lacto-ovo-vegetarians enjoy excellent health."

But health benefits are not the only reason vegetarian diets attract followers.

Certain people, such as Seventh-day Adventists, choose a vegetarian diet because of religious beliefs. Others give up meat because they feel eating animals is unethical. Some believe it's a better use of the Earth's resources to eat low on the food chain—that is, to eat plant foods, rather than the animals that eat the plant foods. And many people eat plant foods simply because they are less expensive than animal foods.

It's wise to take precautions, however, when adopting a diet that entirely excludes animal flesh and dairy products, called a vegan diet.

"The more you restrict your diet, the more difficult it is to get the nutrients you need," says John Vanderveen, Ph.D., director of the Food and Drug Administration's Office of Plant and Dairy Foods and Beverages. "To be healthful, vegetarian diets require very careful, proper planning. Nutrition counseling can help you get started on a diet that is nutritionally adequate."

If appropriately planned, vegan diets, though restrictive, can provide adequate nutrition even for children, according to the American Dietetic Association and the Institute of Food Technologists.

✎ Weird Words

The American Dietetic Association describes three types of vegetarians. They are listed here by the extent to which the diet includes animal foods:

Lacto-Ovo-Vegetarian: Dairy foods and eggs

Lacto-Vegetarian: Dairy foods, but no eggs

Vegan: No animal foods of any type

Plant Food Benefits

Registered dietitian Johanna Dwyer, of Tufts University Medical School and the New England Medical Center Hospital, Boston, summarizes these plant food benefits:

> "Data are strong that vegetarians are at lesser risk for obesity, atonic [reduced muscle tone] constipation, lung cancer, and alcoholism. Evidence is good that risks for hypertension, coronary artery disease, type II diabetes, and gallstones are lower. Data are only fair to poor that risks of breast cancer, diverticular disease of the colon, colonic cancer, calcium kidney stones, osteoporosis, dental erosion, and dental caries are lower among vegetarians."

According to Dwyer, vegetarians' longevity is similar to or greater than that of non-vegetarians, but is influenced in Western countries by vegetarians' "adoption of many healthy lifestyle habits in addition to diet, such as not smoking, abstinence or moderation in the use of alcohol, being physically active, resting adequately, seeking ongoing health surveillance, and seeking guidance when health problems arise."

Can Veggies Prevent Cancer?

The National Cancer Institute, in its booklet *Diet, Nutrition, & Cancer Prevention: A Guide to Food Choices*, states that 35 percent of cancer deaths may be related to diet. The booklet states:

- Diets rich in beta-carotene (the plant form of vitamin A) and vitamin C may reduce the risk of certain cancers.

- Reducing fat in the diet may reduce cancer risk and, in helping weight control, may reduce the risk of heart attacks and strokes.

- Diets high in fiber-rich foods may reduce the risk of cancers of the colon and rectum.

- Vegetables from the cabbage family (cruciferous vegetables) may reduce the risk of colon cancer.

The U.S. Food and Drug Administration (FDA), in fact, authorized several health claims on food labels relating low-fat diets high in some plant-derived foods with a possibly reduced risk of cancer.

While FDA acknowledges that high intakes of fruits and vegetables rich in beta-carotene or vitamin C have been associated with reduced cancer risk, it believes the data are not sufficiently convincing that either nutrient by itself is responsible for the association. Nevertheless, since most fruits and vegetables are low-fat foods and may contain vitamin A (as beta-carotene) and vitamin C, the agency authorized a health claim relating diets low in fat and rich in these foods to a possibly reduced risk of some cancers.

Another claim may relate low-fat diets high in fiber-containing vegetables, fruits, and grains to a possible reduction in cancer risk. (The National Cancer Institute recommends 20 to 30 grams of fiber a day.) Although the exact role of total dietary fiber, fiber components, and other nutrients and substances in these foods is not fully understood, many studies have shown such diets to be associated with reduced risk of some cancers.

Lowering Heart Disease Risk

FDA also notes that diets high in saturated fats and cholesterol increase blood levels of total cholesterol and LDL cholesterol, and thus the risk for coronary heart disease. (The National Cholesterol Education Program recommends a diet with no more than 30 percent fat, of which no more than 10 percent comes from saturated fat.) For this reason, the agency authorized a health claim relating diets low in saturated fat and cholesterol to a possibly reduced risk of coronary heart disease.

Another claim may relate diets low in fat and high in fruits, vegetables, and grain products that contain fiber, particularly soluble fiber, to a possibly reduced risk of coronary heart disease. However, the agency recognizes that it is impossible to adequately distinguish the effects of fiber, including soluble fiber, from those of other food components.

With respect to increasing fiber in the diet, Joanne Slavin, Ph.D., R.D., of the University of Minnesota, in 1990 in *Nutrition Today*, gives this advice:

"The current interest in dietary fiber has allowed recommendations for fiber supplementation to outdistance the scientific research base. Until we have a better understanding of how fiber works its magic, we should recommend to American consumers only a gradual increase in dietary fiber from a variety of sources."

Precautions

The American Dietetic Association's position paper on vegetarian diets states, "Because vegan diets tend to be high in bulk, care should be taken to ensure that caloric intakes are sufficient to meet energy needs, particularly in

---

✔ Quick Tip

Vegetarians who eat no animal products need to be more aware of nutrient sources. Nutrients most likely to be lacking and some non-animal sources are:

- **Vitamin B_{12}:** Fortified soy beverages and cereals

- **Vitamin D:** Fortified soy beverages and sunshine

- **Calcium:** Tofu processed with calcium, broccoli, seeds, nuts, kale, bok choy, legumes (peas and beans), greens, lime-processed tortillas, and soy beverages, grain products, and orange juice enriched with calcium

- **Iron:** Legumes, tofu, green leafy vegetables, dried fruit, whole grains, and iron-fortified cereals and breads, especially whole-wheat. (Absorption is improved by vitamin C, found in citrus fruits and juices, tomatoes, strawberries, broccoli, peppers, dark-green leafy vegetables, and potatoes with skins.)

- **Zinc:** Whole grains (especially the germ and bran), whole-wheat bread, legumes, nuts, and tofu

- **Protein:** Tofu and other soy-based products, legumes, seeds, nuts, grains, and vegetables

infancy and during weaning." Dwyer and Suzanne Havala, also a registered dietitian, updated the paper in the 1993 issue of the association's journal.

It's generally agreed that to avoid intestinal discomfort from increased bulk, a person shouldn't switch to foods with large amounts of fiber all at once. A sensible approach is to slowly increase consumption of grains, legumes, seeds, and nuts. "Some may choose to eliminate red meat but continue to eat fish and poultry occasionally, and such a diet is also to be encouraged," Jack Zeev Yetiv, M.D., Ph.D., in his book *Popular Nutritional Practices: A Scientific Appraisal.*

As with any diet, it's important for the vegetarian diet to include many different foods, since no one food contains all the nutrients required for good health. "The wider the variety, the greater the chance of getting the nutrients you need," says FDA's Vanderveen.

In its position paper on vegetarian diets, the American Dietetic Association states that, with a plant-based daily diet, eating a variety of foods and sufficient calories for energy needs will help ensure adequate intakes of calcium, iron and zinc.

The mixture of proteins from grains, legumes, seeds, nuts, and vegetables provides a complement of amino acids so that deficits in one food are made up by another. Not all types of plant foods need to be eaten at the same meal, since the amino acids are combined in the body's protein pool.

"Soy protein," the paper states, "has been shown to be nutritionally equivalent in protein value to proteins of animal origin and, thus, can serve as the sole source of protein intake if desired."

The Institute of Food Technologists also recommends careful diet planning for vegetarians. This is especially important when the diet excludes dairy foods, to ensure adequate intake of calcium, iron, riboflavin, and vitamin D. For these vegetarians, the institute recommends calcium supplements during pregnancy, when breast-feeding, and for infants and children.

The institute and the American Dietetic Association say a vitamin D supplement may be needed if sunlight exposure is limited. (Sunlight activates a substance in the skin and converts it into vitamin D.)

They also point out that vegan diets should include a reliable source of vitamin B_{12}, because this nutrient occurs only in animal foods. Vitamin B_{12} deficiency can result in irreversible nerve deterioration.

The need for vitamin B_{12} increases during pregnancy, breast-feeding, and periods of growth, Dwyer says. In a recent issue of *Annual Review of Public Health*, she writes that elderly people also should be especially cautious about adopting vegetarian diets because their bodies may absorb vitamin B_{12} poorly.

Unless advised otherwise by a doctor, those taking dietary supplements should limit the dose to 100 percent of the U.S. Recommended Daily Allowances.

With the array of fruits, vegetables, grains, and spices available in U.S. grocery stores and the availability of vegetarian cookbooks, it's easy to devise tasty vegetarian dishes that even non-vegetarians can enjoy.

☞ **Remember!!**

The key to any healthful diet—vegetarian or non-vegetarian—is adherence to sound nutrition principles.

Part 3

Meal Planning

Chapter 22

How To Plan Great Meals

What's your attitude toward healthy eating? Confused by media reports with conflicting information? Concerned but don't want to give up favorite foods? Think healthful foods are boring? Or maybe you think you do eat a healthful diet. Whatever your nutrition attitude, you can make the Food Guide Pyramid work for you.

The "I'm With The Program" Group

You're a member of this group if you try to eat as healthfully as possible. You study food labels and read nutrition articles. Here are some special tips for you:

- Plan meals from the base of the Pyramid up. Start with a grain—pasta or rice, for example—and add one or two vegetables. Next, choose a protein food such as meat, poultry, fish, beans, or eggs. Finish with a fruit or yogurt.

- Size up combination foods according to food groups. Your favorite pizza probably has ingredients from the bread group (crust), vegetable group (tomato sauce, onions, mushrooms), milk group (cheese), and maybe the meat group.

About This Chapter: The text in this chapter is from "How to Plan Great Meals," by Sharon Denny in *Current Health 2*, November 1996 v23 n3 p24(3) © 1996 Weekly Reader Corporation; reprinted with permission.

- When reading labels, check out the serving size. Different products in the same category can have very different portion sizes. For example, a serving of granola might be only 1/4 cup, while a serving of a puffed cereal may be as much as 2 cups.

- Look for more than just fat and calories on food labels. Choose "extra value" foods that contribute to your daily needs for calcium, iron, vitamins A and C, and fiber.

✔ Quick Tip

Use this easy method to keep track of your food choices. Check off each serving of food from the Food Guide Pyramid. If, by dinner time, you are still lacking two vegetables, a meat, two grains, and a milk, you'll know what to eat to complete the day.

If you checked all the boxes, you would get about 2200 calories, the average requirement for teen girls. Teenage boys and very active girls need one or two additional servings in each group to meet their calorie needs.

Grains: Serving size = a slice of bread, 1/2 bun or bagel, 1 ounce cereal, 1/2 cup pasta or rice ❑ ❑ ❑ ❑ ❑ ❑ ❑ ❑ ❑

Vegetables: Serving size = 1/2 cup cooked or diced vegetables, 1 cup leafy greens, or 1/2 cup juice ❑ ❑ ❑

Fruit: Serving size = 1 medium piece of fruit, 3/4 cup juice, or 1/2 cup canned fruit ❑ ❑

Meat and Meat Alternates: Serving size = 2 to 3 ounces lean meat. One ounce lean meat substitutes = 2 tablespoons peanut butter, 1 egg, 1/2 cup beans or tofu ❑ ❑

Milk, Yogurt, Cheese: Serving size = 1 cup milk or yogurt, 1 1/2 ounces cheese ❑ ❑ ❑

The "I Know I Should, But..." Group

If you feel healthful eating takes too much time and means giving up favorite foods, this is your group. You know nutrition is important, but you don't do all you can when it comes to eating healthfully. Your special tips include:

- Use the Food Guide Pyramid as a time saver to plan balanced meals. Make sure that each meal contains foods from at least three of the food groups.

- Keep track of what you eat. Compare your daily diet to the Pyramid guidelines.

- Add variety to your favorite foods by changing just one food group ingredient. Try stir-fried chicken and vegetables with pasta. Use romaine or leaf lettuce in place of iceberg in a tossed salad. Substitute beans for ground beef to make a vegetarian chili.

- Favorite foods can be part of a Pyramid eating plan. A cheeseburger is a meat option. Cookies belong in the bread group, and ice cream fits in with milk, yogurt, and cheese. Just remember to balance higher-fat choices with lower-fat foods.

The "Don't Bother Me" Group

Nutrition seems too complicated, and you're not interested in changing the way you eat. Here are easy tips for your group:

- Take small steps to slowly improve the way you eat. Start by concentrating on just the bread group. Your goal should be to have six or more servings a day from this group. Then move on to the fruit group and work your way up the Pyramid.

- Keep healthy snack foods handy. A fruit, veggie, or yogurt snack can fill in the nutritional gaps in your meals.

- If you eat out often, think about how your meal fits into the Food Guide Pyramid.

It's Not Boring!

Healthful eating doesn't mean boring food! Put these simple tips to work for you, and your meals will be the healthiest and tastiest yet.

- Plan meals ahead of time using the Food Guide Pyramid. Go for variety in all the food groups. Be creative! Use a bagel, tortilla, or pita in place of bread. Explore the taste of new fruits and vegetables. Experiment with different types of cheeses.

- Select foods that complement each other in taste and texture. For example, a baked potato with spicy salsa, crispy stir-fried vegetables with rice, or crunchy apple slices with a peanut butter sandwich.

- Color can make a meal bright and interesting or plain and boring. Simple changes in a one-color meal can make a real difference in its visual appeal. A meal of macaroni and cheese, corn, applesauce, and bread goes from boring to interesting when it becomes macaroni and cheese, peas, fresh apple, and whole-wheat roll.

- Ethnic dishes add variety and new taste sensations to meals. Look for ethnic recipes in cookbooks and magazines. Try seasoning combinations such as basil and garlic, oregano and lemon, or ginger and garlic to liven up plain chicken, pasta, or fish.

- Make healthful menu planning easier by stocking up on nutrient-rich foods.

☞ Remember!!

Go for variety and balance—and you won't have to give up your favorites to have great meals that are great for you.

Chapter 23

Fun and Healthy Recipes

Breakfast

Banana Split Cereal

Who said banana splits were only for dessert? Yogurt, cereal, and fruit combine to make a powerhouse breakfast.

Ingredients

- 1 small, ripe banana
- 1 cup fresh blueberries or other fresh fruit
- 1 cup nonfat or low-fat vanilla yogurt
- 1 cup low-sugar cereal (such as Cheerios, Wheaties, Grape-Nuts, or Bran Flakes)

Directions

1. Peel the banana and slice it lengthwise (from tip to tip). Wash the blueberries by placing them in a colander and running water over them. (If you are using another fruit, wash it and cut it into small pieces.)

2. Spoon the yogurt in a mound in the center of a cereal bowl.

About This Chapter: The recipes in this chapter were taken from "Kitchen Fun for Kids," reprinted with permission. Copyright 2000 Center for Science in the Public Interest (CSPI). Reprinted/Adapted from *Nutrition Action Healthletter*, 1875 Connecticut Ave., N.W., Suite 300, Washington, DC 20009-5728, $24.00 for 10 issues. Additional recipes added as noted from "What Do You Eat," U.S. Department of Agriculture (USDA).

3. Sprinkle the cereal on top of the yogurt.
4. Arrange the banana halves on either side of the yogurt.
5. Sprinkle the top with the blueberries or other fruit.

Per serving: Calories: 279; Total Fat: 2.7 grams (.6 teaspoons); Saturated Fat: 0.5 grams; Sodium: 246 milligrams; Cholesterol: 2 milligrams.

Blueberry Pancakes

Try these berry-licious pancakes on weekend or holiday mornings when you have extra time for breakfast.

Ingredients

- 1 cup all-purpose flour
- 1 cup whole-wheat flour
- 1 teaspoon baking powder
- 1 teaspoon baking soda
- 1 cup buttermilk
- 1 egg
- 1 egg white
- 1 tablespoon vegetable oil
- 1 cup blueberries, fresh or frozen (if frozen there is no need to thaw the berries completely before using them)
- Vegetable spray oil
- Fresh fruit, fruit spread, or light syrup

Directions

1. In a large bowl, mix the flours, baking powder, and baking soda with a wooden spoon (about 10 circles).

2. In a medium bowl, whip the buttermilk, egg, egg white, and oil with a wire whisk until it is fluffy and a light yellow (about 30 quick strokes).

3. Add the wet ingredients to the dry flour mixture. Whip with the wire whisk until it is combined but not smooth (about 20 brisk strokes)—it should be a little bit lumpy.

4. Add the blueberries and gently mix them into the batter using the wooden spoon.

5. Heat a large, nonstick frying pan or griddle to medium-hot (350° F). Spray with vegetable oil spray. Drop a tiny drop of the batter into the frying pan to test for the correct heat—when it sizzles it is ready. Pour

cup of batter into the frying pan. When the pancake is bubbly on top and the edges are starting to brown lightly, carefully flip the pancake using a spatula. Cook on this side for 1 or 2 minutes.

6.   Serve the pancakes immediately, with your favorite fresh fruit, fruit spread, or light syrup.

Per pancake: Calories: 68; Total Fat: 2.1 grams (.5 teaspoons); Saturated Fat: 0.4 grams; Sodium: 103 milligrams; Cholesterol: 24 milligrams.

Lunch

Mental Lentil Tomato Brain Soup

Here's a recipe for a soup you can make after school that will be ready in time for dinner. It takes only 15 to 20 minutes to prepare. Then you can spend 3 hours doing other things and relishing the aroma while the soup simmers.

Ingredients

- 1 pound dried lentils (about 2 and a quarter cups)
- 8 cups water
- 1 large onion, chopped
- 6 carrots, chopped
- 3 stalks celery, chopped
- 1 large can tomatoes, (1 lb., 12 oz. can)
- 1 1/2 teaspoons salt
- 1/2 teaspoon pepper

Optional Seasonings

- 2 bay leaves
- 1 teaspoon sweet basil
- 1 teaspoon thyme

Directions

Put all ingredients and spices, except the tomatoes, into a large pot and simmer for 3 hours. Add more water if the soup gets too thick. Stir in the tomatoes at the end. Makes 11 cups.

Fruit-N-Nut Zamiches

Ingredients

- 1 orange (peeled and cut-up)
- 1 banana (cut into small cubes)
- 1/3 cup of raisins
- 1/3 cup crunchy peanut butter (preferably reduced fat, no sugar, and/or no salt added)
- 8 slices whole-grain bread

Directions

1. Mix the orange, banana, raisins, and peanut butter together in a bowl.

2. Spread the mixture on 4 slices of bread and top with the other 4 slices. This makes a yummy lunch box feast!

Muffin Pizzas

Be a pizza whiz by preparing these miniature pizzas in minutes. Serves 2.

Ingredients

- 2 English muffins (whole wheat if possible)
- 1 small onion
- 4 fresh mushrooms
- 2 tablespoons canned tomato paste, no salt added
- 2 tablespoons water
- 1 teaspoon dried oregano
- black pepper (optional)
- 4 thin slices of part-skim mozzarella cheese

Directions

1. Slice or separate the muffins into halves and place them in a toaster or a toaster oven. Toast until the muffins are golden brown.

2. While the muffins are toasting, cut the ends off of the onion and peel away the outer skin. Chop the onion into little pieces (smaller than a raisin).

3. Wipe mushrooms with a damp paper towel and slice of the very end part of each stem. Slice the mushrooms as thin as you can.

4. Make a tomato sauce by mixing the tomato paste, water, and oregano in a small bowl. Add a dash of black pepper for a spicier pizza.

5. Put your oven mitts on and place the toasted muffins on the broiler pan.

6. Top each with 1 tablespoon of tomato sauce. Sprinkle with onions and mushrooms and place a slice of cheese on top.

7. Put your oven mitts back on and place the pizzas under the broiler (of a stove or a toaster oven), about 4 inches away from the heat. Broil until the cheese melts, about 4 or 5 minutes.

Per pizza: Calories 279; Total Fat: 8.7 grams (2 teaspoons); Saturated Fat: 4.9 grams; Sodium: 447 milligrams; Cholesterol: 23 milligrams.

Tabouleh

This recipe from the USDA makes 13 servings.

Ingredients

- 1-1/2 cups bulgur wheat (No. 3 size)
- 1-1/2 cups boiling water
- 3 cups fresh tomatoes, diced
- 1/4 cup fresh cucumber, peeled, seeded, and diced
- 1/4 cup fresh parsley, chopped
- 1/4 cup plus 2 tbsp onions, minced
- 2 tsp fresh mint, chopped, or 1/4 Tsp dried
- 1/4 tsp cumin (optional)
- 1 tsp salt
- 1/4 cup lemon juice
- 2 tbsp vegetable oil

Directions

1. Combine bulgur and boiling water. Let stand for 30 minutes or until water is absorbed. Do not drain.

2. Add the tomatoes, cucumbers, parsley, onions, mint and cumin (optional) to the bulgur and stir to blend.

3. In a small bowl, combine the salt and lemon juice. Slowly whisk in oil.

4. Add dressing to salad, and toss to coat all ingredients. Serve chilled!

Per Serving: 91 Calories; 3 g Protein; 16g Carbohydrate; 2.5 g Total Fat; 4 g Fiber

Dinner

Super Stir-Fry

When preparing this dish, keep all of the vegetables that you are slicing in separate piles since you will be adding them to the wok at different times. Serves 4.

This oriental way to cook is healthy because you use a small amount of fat and cook vegetables for a short time, which helps preserve their nutrients. The tofu is rich in protein and is a substitute for chicken or beef. Remember to use reduced-sodium soy sauce.

Ingredients

- 2 garlic cloves
- 2 large stalks broccoli
- 3 carrots, about 5 inches long
- 6 to 8 fresh mushrooms
- 1 medium-size green pepper
- 1 medium-sized onion

- 1 teaspoon peanut oil
- 1 tablespoon water
- 1 tablespoon mild or low-sodium soy sauce
- Firm tofu, cut into small cubes to make 3/4 cup.

Directions

1. Peel the garlic and force it through a garlic press. Set aside. (If you don't have a garlic press, then just chop the garlic into tiny pieces.)

2. Wash the broccoli and cut off the florets.

3. Peel the carrots, cut off the tops and bottoms, and slice the carrots into coined-shaped pieces.

4. Wipe the mushrooms with a damp paper towel and cut off the end part of each stem. Slice the mushrooms into pieces to make 1 cup.

5. Cut the green pepper in half lengthwise and remove the stem and seeds. Wash the halves and cut them into small strips (about 1 inch long and inch wide).

6. Cut the ends off the onions and peel the outer skin. Slice the onion into thick disks, then separate into rings.

7. In a wok or frying pan, heat the oil on medium-high heat.

8. Add the garlic and onion and stir with a wooden spoon for 15 seconds.

9. Stir in the broccoli florets, carrots, and green pepper.

10. Add the water. Cover the pan and cook until the vegetables are about half-done, about 6 minutes.

11. Add soy sauce and stir well with the wooden spoon.

12. Stir in the mushrooms and tofu and cook for another 5 minutes. Serve immediately. Try eating this meal with chopsticks instead of forks!

Per serving: Calories: 116; Total Fat 3.9 grams (.9 teaspoons); Saturated Fat: 0.5; Sodium: 214 milligrams; Cholesterol: 0 milligrams.

Fabulous Fish Sticks

Forget those rock-hard sticks in the freezer—try this recipe and do it yourself. Serves 4.

Ingredients

- 1 pound boneless, skinless cod
- 1 egg white
- 1/4 cup skim milk
- 3 to 4 slices dry bread
- 1 teaspoon black pepper
- 1 teaspoon dried parsley
- 1/4 teaspoon paprika
- 1 lemon, cut into wedges

Directions

1. Preheat the oven to 475° F.

2. Cut the fish into 8 stick-shaped pieces. Try to make them as equal in size as possible.

3. Combine the egg and milk in a small bowl and briskly whip with a fork or wire whisk until foamy (about 15 quick strokes).

4. Place the bread in a [zipper-closing styled] plastic bag. Close the bag and crush the bread into fine crumbs by rolling over it with the rolling

pin. Measure out 1 cup of crumbs. With your fingers, mix together the bread crumbs, pepper, parsley, and paprika on a dinner plate.

5. Dip the fish into the egg mixture, coat with the crumb mixture, and place the fish in a nonstick baking dish (if using a regular baking dish, lightly grease bottom with vegetable oil so the fish will not stick during cooking). Repeat this procedure until all the fish is breaded, then squeeze lemon juice evenly over the fish sticks.

6. Put your oven mitts on, open the oven door, and place the dish in the middle of the center rack. Set timer and bake the fish sticks for 20 minutes.

7. Serve with your favorite green vegetable and a baked potato.

Per serving: Calories: 201; Total Fat: 2.1 grams (.5 teaspoons); Saturated Fat: 0.5 grams; Sodium: 266 milligrams; Cholesterol: 51 milligrams.

Sweet Potatoes With Lime

This recipe from the USDA makes 8 servings.

Ingredients

- 4 sweet potatoes, washed
- juice of 2 limes
- 3-4 cilantro leaves (optional)
- 1/4 tsp salt (optional)

Directions

1. Preheat the oven to 375° F.

2. Take a fork and poke a few holes in each sweet potato. Bake the sweet potatoes whole in their skins, until tender, about 45 minutes to 1 hour.

3. When the potatoes are tender, slit open the skin and scoop out the flesh onto a serving dish. Season with salt (optional).

5. Squeeze fresh lime juice over the top, and sprinkle with 3 or 4 cilantro leaves (optional).

Per Serving: 61 Calories; 1 g Protein; 15g Carbohydrate; .1 g Total Fat; 2 g Fiber

Dessert

Berry Pops

Fruit-sicles are a great treat on a hot summer day. Serves 12.

Homemade is better! Most ice pops are made from water, sugar, artificial colors, and artificial flavors. These pops are made with real fruit.

Ingredients

- 1 cup of berry juice blend, such as cranberry-raspberry, boysenberry, or apple-raspberry
- 1 tablespoon (1 envelope) unflavored gelatin
- 2 cups nonfat or low-fat vanilla yogurt
- 1 cup frozen, unsweetened berries (blueberries, strawberries, raspberries or blackberries)

Special Tools

- 12 wooden sticks (available at most supermarkets and craft stores)
- 12 four-ounce paper cups
- aluminum foil

Directions

1. Place the juice in a pan and sprinkle the gelatin over it. Cook over low heat, stirring constantly with a wooden spoon until the gelatin crystals disappear. Using a pot holder and both hands, remove the pan from the heat and place on a hot pad.

2. In a blender or food processor, mix the yogurt, berries and warm gelatin mixture. Blend until smooth (about 2 minutes).

3. Place the paper cups on a cookie sheet (one that will fit in the freezer). Fill the cups with the blended mixture and place a sheet of aluminum foil over the tops of the cups.

4. Insert the stick for each pop by making a slit in the foil with a knife over the center of each cup and placing the stick into the cup. The aluminum foil will help keep the stick in place.

5.   Place the tray in the freezer and freeze until hard.

6.   Remove the pops from the cups by peeling away the paper.

Per berry pop: Calories: 42; Total Fat: less than 1 gram; Saturated Fat: 0.1; Sodium: milligrams; Cholesterol: 0 milligrams.

Fruit Yogurt Shake

This recipe from the USDA makes 2 servings.

Ingredients

- 1 cup fruit (peaches, strawberries, bananas) cut up
- 4 scoops (1 and 1/3 cups) non-fat frozen yogurt
- 2 cups skim milk, ice cold
- 2 tbsp sugar

Directions

1.   Cut up the fruit—carefully. Put all the ingredients in a blender, close the top, then puree.

2.   Pour the mixture into two chilled glasses, and serve with a straw. Cool!

Per serving: 291 Calories; 12 g Protein; 53 g Carbohydrate; 0.6 g Total Fat; 1 g Fiber

Fresh Fruit Kabobs
With Chocolate Sauce

This recipe from the USDA makes 6 Servings.

Ingredients

- 12 strawberries
- 24 melon balls (honeydew, cantaloupe)
- 6 ounces angel food cake, cut into 1-inch cubes
- 1-1/3 cups semi-sweet chocolate chips
- 1 tbsp lowfat buttermilk (or lowfat milk)
- 6 wooden skewers

Directions

1. Wash the strawberries, and pick off the stems. With a melon baller or small spoon, make the melon balls.

2. Carefully cut the cake into one inch squares.

3. Arrange fruit and cake on the wooden skewers. The pattern is up to you! Place the skewered fruit sticks on a serving plate.

4. Melt the chocolate chips and milk together over low heat.

5. Pour the warm sauce over the fruit sticks, turning them over to cover completely. Let them cool a moment. Enjoy!

Per Serving: 354 Calories; 5 g Protein; 63g Carbohydrate; 12.6 g Total Fat; 7 g Fiber

Chapter 24

The Best And Worst Breakfasts

Among The Worst

- fatty sweets (danish, doughnuts, cinnamon rolls)
- fatty, salty meats (sausage, bacon, ham), and
- eggs (whose yolks add more cholesterol to the average American's diet than any other single food).

Among The Best

- fresh fruit (oranges, bananas, berries) or juice
- dairy foods (low-fat milk, yogurt), and
- whole grains (whole-grain hot or cold cereals, whole-wheat toast).

Popular Breakfast Items

The trouble is that the food industry keeps tempting us with new worsts.

"Dessert for breakfast is a trend that we have been following for several years," Eleanor Hanson of Foodwatch recently told *Restaurants & Institutions* magazine. Foodwatch is an Edina, Minnesota, consulting firm that analyzes food trends.

About This Chapter: This chapter contains text from "The Best and Worst Breakfasts," compiled by Ingrid VanTuinen and "Great Breakfast Grab-and Go's," both reprinted with permission. Copyright 2000 Center for Science in the Public Interest (CSPI). Reprinted/ Adapted from *Nutrition Action Healthletter*, 1875 Connecticut Ave., N.W., Suite 300, Washington, DC 20009-5728. $24.00 for 10 issues.

"We're seeing streusel in cereal, chocolate in muffins and scones, and monster-size cinnamon rolls. Blurring is occurring on the sweets continuum."

People who think twice about having a DoveBar for dessert might not suspect that an Almond Croissant from Au Bon Pain is worse than two DoveBars. Do you really want to "grab and go" 630 calories, nearly a day's worth of artery-clogging fat, and five teaspoons of sugar?

Another trend: mega-sandwiches. McDonald's new bagel sandwiches have at least double the fat and calories of its pioneering Egg McMuffin. And its Spanish Omelet Bagel has more fat and calories than a Big Mac or a Quarter Pounder with Cheese.

We examined popular breakfast items from fast-food chains, sit-down restaurants, and supermarkets. Most of the numbers came from the manufacturers. When their information fell short, we sent a handful of items— from places like Au Bon Pain, Dunkin' Donuts, and Einstein Bros Bagels— to an independent laboratory for analysis.

The results should sound a wake-up call. If restaurant foods came with the same "Nutrition Facts" labels you can read on, say, the back of a cereal box, the lines at Dunkin' Donuts might be a lot shorter.

Cereal

The more you look at the breakfasts people eat outside the home, the better cereal looks. True, some cereals are more than a third sugar and are mostly—or all—refined flour plus a quarter of a vitamin pill. And that list includes not just kids-only brands but cereals like General Mills' Frosted Wheaties. But even those low-fiber "candy cereals" are relatively low in calories (about 120 per serving) and fat (assuming you eat them with one percent or skim milk).

High-fiber, whole-grain, low-sugar cereals like shredded wheat, Wheaties, or bran flakes make a top-notch breakfast, especially if you add fresh fruit. No other breakfast offers so much fiber, calcium, and other nutrients for so few calories and so little fat.

If you're eating at the office ("deskfast"), bring cereal and plain low-fat yogurt (if milk is too messy) in a plastic container. It should only take a minute to slice in a banana or throw on some blueberries.

Caution: Don't confuse cereal with cereal bars. The bars may be low in fat and fortified with vitamins, but they're not high in whole grains or fiber, and people are less likely to eat them with low-fat milk or fresh fruit. While the fruit splashed over the ads and labels looks good, it's the equivalent of a generous swipe of jam on a slice of mostly white bread.

Eggs

It's not just the eggs that make egg breakfasts so fatty. It's the fat they're cooked in, the sausage or cheese in the omelet, and what comes on the side. Most people who eat eggs for breakfast have them with something else. And that something is often buttered toast, hash browns, sausage, bacon, biscuits, or a croissant.

That's why a McDonald's Big Breakfast (scrambled eggs, sausage, hash browns, and a biscuit) or a Denny's Grand Slam (eggs, sausage, bacon, and pancakes) supplies three-quarters of a day's fat and saturated fat. And that's why a Denny's Slim Slam (Egg Beaters, pancakes with fruit topping, and grilled ham) does away with three-quarters of the fat in the Grand Slam—largely by replacing what comes on the side.

Of course, fast-food chains are now happy to serve you eggs-to-go…on a bagel, croissant, biscuit, or English muffin. And they pile on enough sausage, ham, cheese, and cooking grease to make sure that you get the equivalent of a burger or worse.

Muffins

Our appetite for muffins grew by 25 percent from 1987 to 1996. That's not all that grew. Entenmann's still sells 2½-ounce Blueberry Muffins. But McDonald's and Dunkin' Donuts' muffins approach four ounces, and the muffins at Au Bon Pain come closer to five. That means calories in the 300 to 500 range, ten to 20 grams of fat, and five to ten teaspoons of total sugars (including the sugar from the berries or other fruit).

The good news is that the fat in muffins is less of a threat to your arteries than the fat in doughnuts, danish, and croissants. Only two to four grams per muffin are saturated or trans fat (exception: Dunkin's Chocolate Chip Muffin hits six).

Another plus: McDonald's, Dunkin' Donuts (though not at every outlet), and Au Bon Pain all sell low-fat muffins that trim the calories to 250 to 300 and the fat to no more than three or four grams. And all sell bran muffins with at least three grams of fiber, so you get some of the bran's phytochemicals and nutrients. But you're still talking about mostly white flour and sugar for breakfast.

Doughnuts

All doughnuts are not created equal.

"Cake" doughnuts can have twice as much fat as "yeast" doughnuts. And a chocolate or coconut coating or frosting is worse than other coatings, whether it's yeast or cake.

Take a Glazed or Sugar Raised yeast donut at Dunkin' Donuts. Eat only one (good luck!) and you can get away with about 200 calories, a teaspoon or two of sugar, and eight or 12 grams of fat.

That's not terrific. Like any doughnut, the trans fat in the frying shortening matches the damage caused by the saturated fat. We found six grams—

✔ Quick Tip

If you are having a bagel for breakfast, consider using fruit preserves instead of cream cheese. If you must put cream cheese on your bagel, try:

- fat-free cream cheese,

- "light" cream cheese, which has half the fat of regular cream cheese, or

- "double whipped" cream cheese, which has at least a quarter less fat than regular (non-whipped) cream cheese.

nearly a third of a day's worth—of "bad" fat (saturated plus trans) in one yeast Glazed Donut. But you could do a lot worse.

A single Dunkin' Donuts Chocolate Cake Glazed Donut, for example, has 340 calories, three teaspoons of sugar, and 22 grams of fat—12 of them trans or saturated. Of course, doughnut lovers seldom stop at one.

Dunkin' makes it tough by running frequent promotions like "Buy six, get six free." And don't let your eyes wander over to the crullers, fritters, or coffee rolls while you're waiting in line. Think of each as 250 to 300 calories of deep-fried sugar-coated flour.

Bagels

You can't talk about bagels without talking about cream cheese. And it's the cream cheese that can turn a decent breakfast into a lousy one.

Unless you get whole-wheat or multi-grain, your bagel is essentially three to five one-ounce slices of white bread. That typically means about 250 to 350 calories, little or no fat or sugar, and 500 to 700 mg of sodium. (A few varieties, like chocolate chip, cheese, or nut, might hit four to seven grams of fat.)

While you may not be getting whole grains or fruit in a bagel-only breakfast, you're also not getting a load of fried fat and/or sugar, like you would with a doughnut, danish, croissant, or muffin.

Then there's the shmear. At Dunkin' Donuts, the largest bagel-seller in the country, a plain bagel with (regular) cream cheese has 540 calories and 19 grams of fat, 12 of them saturated—more than half a day's worth. Who knew? And don't think you're getting much protein from the cream cheese. It's more cream than cheese.

In contrast, at most Einstein Bros locations, all the cream cheeses are "double whipped," which means they have at least a quarter less fat than regular (non-whipped) cream cheese. And eight of the 11 flavors have half the fat of regular cream cheese. (Those eight are labeled "25 percent reduced fat"—don't ask us why Einstein doesn't call them "50 percent reduced fat" or "light.")

Solution: At home, if you're not willing to go naked or use fat-free cream cheese, try preserves, tub margarine, or a thin layer of light cream cheese (it's got half the fat of regular). Outside, if it's gotta be cream cheese, make sure you get Einstein's 25% reduced fat or Au Bon Pain's or Dunkin' Donuts' lite (they both have half the fat of regular)…and get it on the side, so you can use a thin layer.

Cream cheese used to be the worst thing you could do to a bagel. No longer. The new bagel sandwiches make cream cheese look good.

Breakfast Sandwiches

Burger King's most popular breakfast item is the Croissan'wich. Each day, the number-two chain dispatches more than 800,000 to coronary arteries across the nation. Leave it to BK to combine all three of the worst breakfast foods—pastry, sausage, and egg—into one cheap, hold-in-your-hand package. Now you can gobble up 500-some calories and

> ### ✣ It's A Fact!!
> Some fast food breakfast sandwiches and hash brown products contain as many calories and as much fat as their chains' cheeseburgers.

more than half a day's bad fat and cholesterol while you wait at a traffic light.

Maybe Burger King's recent success inspired McDonald's, Dunkin' Donuts, and Einstein Bros to create their bagel sandwiches. Most will run you 500 to 600 calories and half a day's fat, sat fat, and sodium. That's like eating a Big Mac. Missing are the fruit, low-fat milk, and high-fiber whole grains that many people eat at breakfast—or not at all.

Cinnamon Rolls

Like muffins, cinnamon rolls are, well, on a roll, climbing 25 percent between 1987 and 1996. They're nothing more than breakfast cake.

But at least when you buy Pillsbury Cinnamon Rolls at the supermarket, there's a chance that you'll eat only one, which means 150 calories, five grams of fat, and two teaspoons of sugar. Move up to Pillsbury Grands and the numbers double. But that's still better than the Cini-minis Pillsbury makes for Burger King.

With icing, your "mini" fast-food breakfast totals 530 calories, nine teaspoons of sugar, and 22 grams of fat, nine of them saturated or trans. Cini-minis have doubled Burger King's breakfast sales. What's next? Cini-minis with chocolate coating, M&M's, and Reese's Pieces?

French Toast

At home, you can make delicious French toast with whole-wheat bread, low-fat milk, and Egg Beaters. With Burger King's French Toast Sticks you get white bread and enough sugar and frying grease to supply 500 calories and half a day's "bad" fat. And the company sells over 165 million sticks a year.

Hash Browns

Potatoes are the most frequently ordered breakfast food in restaurants. Fast-food hash browns are fattier than fries. And Burger King's are fattier than McDonald's. Fatwise, a small order of Burger King's Hash Brown Rounds is like the chain's Bacon Cheeseburger. And a large order means 70 percent more fat to line your arteries, which brings us to…

The Best And Worst Chains

Between its hash browns, French Toast Sticks, Croissan'wiches, and Cini-minis, Burger King deserves special recognition for its efforts to block Americans' arteries before they get to work. It wins our coveted "Breakfast Busters" award. Bypass Burger King before you need your own bypass.

In contrast, Einstein Bros deserves a "Breakfast Boosters" award for switching to lower-fat cream cheese. We've still got plenty of bones to pick with its menu. But eight flavors of lower-fat cream cheese—from cappuccino to jalapeño salsa—is a trend we'd like to see spread.

Great Breakfast "Grab-and-Go's"

Who needs cream cheese and croissants? Skip the Cini-minis and cereal bars. Making your own healthy grab-and-go breakfast is a snap. Here are a handful of ideas to get you started. You can probably think of dozens of variations. If you're still hungry, add a banana, apple, or other fruit to the menu. Each grab-and-go tip has no more than 400 calories, 8 grams of fat (3 of them saturated), and 570 milligrams of sodium.

- Scoop 1/2 cup low-fat cottage cheese into a cantaloupe or honeydew half.

- Add fresh fruit or cereal (like raisin bran or low-fat granola) to plain low-fat or non-fat yogurt.

- Layer a whole-grain toaster waffle with 1/2 cup plain low-fat yogurt and 1/2 cup berries.

- Spread 2 Tbs. of hummus on half a pumpernickel bagel.

- Combine 1/4 cup low-fat ricotta cheese with 1/2 cup apple sauce and a dash of cinnamon. Sprinkle with Grape-Nuts.

- Stir 1/2 cup each of plain low-fat yogurt and orange-pineapple-banana juice with 1/3 cup of sliced banana and 1/2 dozen fresh or frozen blueberries. Freeze overnight.

- Blend 1/2 cup each of plain low-fat yogurt and orange juice with 1/2 frozen banana and a few frozen strawberries.

> **☞ Remember!!**
>
> Many popular breakfast items contain as much fat and sugar as dessert items. For healthier options, consider fresh fruit, low-fat dairy foods, and whole grain products, such as whole-grain hot or cold cereals, whole-wheat toast, or whole grain bagels.

- Spread 1 Tbs. peanut butter on whole-wheat bread and wrap it around a banana.

- Melt 1 thin slice of Jarlsberg Lite Swiss Cheese over sliced tomato on an English muffin.

- Stuff half a whole-wheat pita with 1/2 cup low-fat cottage cheese and sliced peaches, pears, or banana.

- Top a raisin bagel with fat-free cream cheese (or a *thin* layer of "lite") and thin apple slices.

- Roll a tortilla up with scrambled Egg Beaters and salsa.

Chapter 25

Sandwiches: Can You Tell The Good Guys From The Bad?

The suspects are lined up. Can you tell the good guys from the bad?

We're all familiar with "The Line-Up" from countless TV shows and movies. The cops have their suspect, the witness is ready to make an ID, and a motley cast of characters lines up. As viewers, it's often tough to tell the good guys from the bad. We look for one subtle clue to tip us off. The shifty eyes. The fidgety hands. The guy wearing the striped prison garb.

At first glance, selecting a healthy sandwich might feel like the same process. Who's really the good guy—the sandwich that will satisfy yet still be healthy and nutritious—and which one is a heart attack on rye? Most sandwiches, if fixed properly, can be healthy and nutritious, says Carmen Conrey, a registered dietitian at the Johns Hopkins Weight Management Center.

Condiment Crimes

The first rule of thumb, when making or buying a sandwich, is to watch what you add to it, says Conrey. Slathering on mayo is an easy way to send fat and calorie content skyrocketing. Salad dressings such as Thousand Island and blue cheese do the same. You can take control by selecting low-fat or no-fat condiments. If you're ordering at a deli or restaurant and there are

The Sandwich Line-Up

Food	Calories (grams)	Fat (milligrams)	Sodium
Ham and Cheese (5 ounces boiled ham; 1 slice American cheese)	370	14	2080
Ham and Cheese (6 slices Healthy Choice ham = 2 ounces; 1 slice Kraft fat-free American cheese)	290	5	1190
Turkey (4 ounces deli turkey)	370	7	490
Tuna Salad (1 ready-mix can)	130	8	920
Peanut Butter and Jelly (2 tablespoons peanut butter and 1 tablespoon jelly)	440	20	570
Cold Cuts Sub (6" Subway Italian BMT)	460	22	1660
Egg Salad (2 eggs and 2 tablespoons mayonnaise)	550	36	700
Chicken Salad (2.5 ounces chicken and 3 tablespoons mayonnaise)	610	39	710
Chicken Salad (2.5 ounces chicken and 2 tablespoons fat-free mayonnaise)	330	6	710
BLT (2 ounces bacon = 5 strips; lettuce and tomato)	540	32	1330
Bagel and Cream Cheese	400	12	670

no low-fat options available, ask for your condiments on the side. That way you control how much you use. Finally, keep an eye on ketchup and barbecue sauce if you're watching sodium intake.

Some people think mayo and salad dressings are the only flavorful toppings out there. Conrey suggests adding onions, tomatoes, sprouts, green peppers, pickles, mushrooms, cucumbers and different types of lettuce. This will "beef up" the sandwich and add fiber and flavor without calories. With all this added flavor, you'll be less likely to pile on mayo and cheese. If you can't live without mayo's consistency or think a sandwich without some dressing is just too dry, try a mayo alternative like hummus or mustard.

> ✎ **Weird Words**
>
> Condiment: An item served with or on food, usually salty or spicy. Examples include pickles and catsup.
>
> Hummus: A sandwich spread or dip made from pureed chick peas.

Meaty Misdemeanors

If you've been eating lean meats at the dinner table, you can do the same with deli meats. A lot of delis post the fat content, says Conrey. Look for labels or signs that read "30 percent or less from fat." If you're selecting pre-packaged lunchmeats, choose those that contain 3 grams of fat for every 100 calories. As for sodium content, stick to less than 300 milligrams.

Selecting leaner cheeses can also help make your sandwich healthier and more nutritious. One rule of thumb is that white cheeses tend to be a little lower in fat and calories than yellow cheeses. Part-skim mozzarella is a great option, as are many of the fat-free or reduced-fat cheeses on the market today. Leave off just one slice of cheddar cheese and save 110 calories and 9 grams of mostly saturated fat!

Law-Abiding Bread

If you've been steering clear of sandwiches because you think the bread makes them fattening, think again. Most breads are not really fattening, says Conrey. So sidle on up to the deli counter and have a go. When you do, choosing whole-wheat or whole- grain bread will help make your sandwich more nutritious. Avoid ever-tempting, oh-so-tasty croissants. Aside from those, everything else is pretty much low fat.

Fat Offenders: Salad Sandwiches

The big culprits for high fat content in the sandwich category are the salads—things such as tuna, chicken, and egg salad. Because of the mayonnaise content, these favorites can be loaded with fat and calories. If you're eating out or ordering at the deli, it's probably best to avoid these. That doesn't mean you have to avoid them altogether, though. Making your own at home with lower quantities of fat-free mayo can do the trick. Substituting 3 tablespoons of regular mayo with 2 tablespoons of fat-free mayo can bring down the calories in a tuna salad sandwich from 580 to 310. The same change slashes the fat content from 38 grams to a mere 5!

☞ Remember!!

The bottom line is that by making a few informed choices, sandwiches don't have to be villains of good health. There are as many healthful options as there are items on a New York deli's chalkboard. "A lot of people get stuck on turkey as the only healthy alternative," says Conrey. "But if you know what to choose, other things can be equally healthy."

Chapter 26

Smart Snacking For Teens On The Go

Between running to class, homework, sports, babysitting, and dating . . . who has time to eat healthy? And when you do stop to eat, it may be tempting to grab a burger and fries or potato chips and candy. Even though your schedule is hectic, healthy eating can supply the fuel you need to keep you going. But if you don't have time to eat three well-balanced meals a day, what's the answer? One word: snacks. Read this chapter to find out how eating small, nutritious meals throughout the day can keep your energy level high and your mind alert, without taking up a lot of your time.

Why Healthy Snacking Is Good For You

Snacking can be a great way to get all the vitamins and nutrients your growing body needs. You may be noticing that your body is demanding more food all the time; it may seem like you can never get enough to eat! This is perfectly normal as you go through puberty.

Small, healthy meals are terrific for satisfying that nagging hunger. But you need to pay attention to what you're eating. Gobbling down a large order of fries after class may give you a temporary boost but a high-fat snack will only slow you down in the long run. To keep your energy levels going consistently, look for foods that contain complex carbohydrates like bagels, graham crackers, or unsweetened cereal and foods that contain protein such as low-fat yogurt and skim milk.

Snacking every 3 to 4 hours will help keep you going when full meals just aren't feasible. Toss some fruit or low-fat granola bars in your backpack so you won't feel tempted to buy fast food or unhealthy vending machine snacks when the munchies hit. Remember there is no substitute for breakfast or some form of nutrition within 2 hours of getting up. A bagel on the way out the door or an apple in the hallway between classes is far better than nothing at all.

Choosing Tasty Snacks

Snacking doesn't have to be boring as long as you have a variety of
choices. Low-fat pretzels and spicy
mustard or flavored rice cakes
topped with jam are tasty and easy.
Instead of corn chips, try baked tortilla chips. Instead of ice cream, try non-
fat frozen yogurt or fruit sherbet. Salsa can

> ♣ **It's A Fact!!**
>
> The average American eats
> about 147 pounds of
> sugars a year.

take the place of cheese- or sour cream-based dips and lowfat angel food cake is a yummy substitute for pound cake. And if you're in a rush, a glass of 100% juice or skim milk is a good source of quick calories.

What Does "Healthy" Really Mean?

Choosing healthy snacks means being cautious of food labels that make false or questionable claims. Many food manufacturers are now labeling their products with words like "all natural" and "pure." This doesn't mean that the foods are nutritious. A food may contain all natural ingredients but may still be high in fat. A good example is granola bars. If you're craving something sweet to munch on, you may think it's better to choose the granola bar over a chocolate bar. Although a granola bar may be a good source of certain vitamins and nutrients, it may also contain a surprisingly large amount of fat.

On average, about 35% of the calories in a granola bar come from fat, unless the granola bars are of the low-fat variety—check the package to be sure.

Smart Snacking Strategies

Becoming a healthy snacker will take small adjustments in your eating habits. Try taking a snack break with a friend; by taking time with your bud, you can help to remind each other to catch up on skipped meals. Stash some fruit, pretzels, or baby carrots in your backpack or workout bag so you always have something nearby.

Evenings can be a tempting time for indulging in fatty, sugary snacks. Don't ignore these cravings—if you're hungry, your body is probably telling you that it needs nutrients. The trick is to pick the right snacks to fill the hunger gap. Fig bars, rice cakes, or air-popped popcorn are just a few good choices.

Treats To Try

Here are some healthy snacks to try:

- Ants on a log—spread nut butter on celery sticks and top with raisins.

- Banana ice cream—peel several very ripe bananas, break into 1-inch pieces and freeze in a sealed plastic bag until very hard. Just before serving, run through a juicer or blender with a small amount of water or juice. Serve immediately. Add berries for a different flavor or top with fruit or nuts.

- Mini pizzas—spoon pizza sauce onto a bagel. Top with low-fat mozzarella cheese and your favorite veggies and toast or bake at low setting until cheese is melted and bagel is crispy.

- Healthy popsicles—freeze fresh, unsweetened juice in popsicle makers or ice cube trays.

- Low-fat pita and hummus—warm pita in oven on low setting and cut into small triangles. Dip in a tasty, low-fat hummus. Hummus is available in yummy flavors like garlic and spicy red pepper.

✔ **Quick Tip**

How can you snack smart? Be choosy! Pick a variety of foods from these groups:

- *Fresh fruits and raw vegetables*
- berries
- oranges
- grapefruit
- melons
- pineapple
- pears
- tangerines
- broccoli
- celery
- carrots
- cucumbers
- tomatoes
- unsweetened fruit and veg- etable juices
- canned fruits in natural juices

- *Grains*
- bread
- plain bagels
- unsweetened cereals
- unbuttered popcorn
- tortilla chips (baked, not fried)

- *Grains, continued*
- pretzels (low-salt)
- pasta
- plain crackers

- *Milk and dairy products*
- low or non-fat milk
- low or non-fat yogurt
- low or non-fat cheeses
- low or non-fat cottage cheese

- *Meat, nuts, and seeds*
- chicken
- turkey
- sliced meats
- pumpkin seeds
- sunflower seeds
- nuts

- *Others*: these snacks combine foods from the different groups
- pizza
- tacos

Snack Smart For Healthy Teeth

What's Wrong With Sugary Snacks, Anyway?

Sugary snacks taste so good—but they aren't so good for your teeth or your body. The candies, cakes, cookies, and other sugary foods that kids love to eat between meals can cause tooth decay. Some surgary foods have a lot of fat in them too.

Kids who consume sugary snacks eat many different kinds of sugar every day, including table sugar (sucrose) and corn sweeteners (fructose). Starchy snacks can also break down into sugars once they're in your mouth.

Did you know that the average American eats about 147 pounds of sugars a year? That's a big pile of sugar! No wonder the average 17-year-old in this country has more than three decayed teeth!

How Do Sugars Attack Your Teeth?

Invisible germs called bacteria live in your mouth all the time. Some of these bacteria form a sticky material called plaque on the surface of the teeth. When you put sugar in your mouth, the bacteria in the plaque gobble up the sweet stuff and turn it into acids. These acids are powerful enough to dissolve the hard enamel that covers your teeth. That's how cavities get started. If you don't eat much sugar, the bacteria can't produce as much of the acid that eats away enamel.

How Can I "Snack Smart" To Protect Myself From Tooth Decay?

Before you start munching on a snack, ask yourself what's in the food you've chosen. Is it loaded with sugar? If it is, think again. Another choice would be better for your teeth. And keep in mind that certain kinds of sweets can do more damage than others. Gooey or chewy sweets spend more time sticking to the surface of your teeth. Because sticky snacks stay in your mouth longer than foods that you quickly chew and swallow, they give your teeth a longer sugar bath.

You should also think about when and how often you eat snacks. Do you nibble on sugary snacks many times throughout the day, or do you usually just have dessert after dinner? Damaging acids form in your mouth every time you eat a sugary snack. The acids continue to affect your teeth for at least 20 minutes before they are neutralized and can't do any more harm. So, the more times you eat sugary snacks during the day, the more often you feed bacteria the fuel they need to cause tooth decay.

If you eat sweets, it's best to eat them as dessert after a main meal instead of several times a day between meals. Whenever you eat sweets—in any meal or snack—brush your teeth well with a fluoride toothpaste afterward.

Deciding About Snacks

When you're deciding about snacks, think about:

- the number of times a day you eat sugary snacks
- how long the sugary food stays in your mouth
- the texture of the sugary food (chewy? sticky?)

If you snack after school, before bedtime, or other times during the day, choose something without a lot of sugar or fat. There are lots of tasty, filling snacks that are less harmful to your teeth—and the rest of your body—than foods loaded with sugars and low in nutritional value.

Low-fat choices like raw vegetables, fresh fruits, or whole-grain crackers or bread are smart choices. Eating the right foods can help protect you from tooth decay and other diseases.

☞ Remember!!

Snacking can be a great way to get all the vitamins and nutrients your growing body needs. But you need to pay attention to what you're eating. To keep your energy levels going consistently, look for foods that contain complex carbohydrates like bagels, graham crackers, or unsweetened cereal and foods that contain protein such as low-fat yogurt and skim milk.

- Choose sugary foods less often.

- Avoid sweets between meals.

- Eat a variety of low or non-fat foods from the basic groups.

- Brush your teeth with fluoride toothpaste after snacks and meals.

Chapter 27

What Every Teen Chef Should Know About Food Safety

You have your recipe, your ingredients, your apron, the whole deal. But before you start slicing and dicing, do you know how to prepare food safely? This means more than keeping your hands away from a whirring blade—it means knowing how to avoid spreading bacteria, knowing tips for safe shopping, and more.

Why Food Safety Matters

You might think that as long as food looks OK, it doesn't really matter how it's been prepared. But food that hasn't been prepared safely may contain bacteria like *E. coli*. Unsafe food can also spread foodborne illnesses like salmonellosis (pronounced: sal-moan-ell-oh-sis) and campylobacter (pronounced: cam-pie-low-bak-ter) infection. (Even the names sound gross!) The good news is you can keep on top of bacteria and foodborne illness by playing it safe when buying, preparing, and storing food.

Start At The Supermarket

You have your shopping list in one hand and that shopping cart with the bad wheel in the other. But where should you start and how do you know which foods are safe? Take a peek at these tips:

- Make sure you put refrigerated foods in your cart last. For example, meat, fish, eggs, and milk should hit your cart after cereals, produce, and chips.

- When buying packaged meat, poultry (chicken or turkey), or fish, check the expiration date on the label (the date may be printed on the front, side, or bottom, depending on the food). Don't buy a food if it has expired.

- Don't buy fish or meat that has a strong or strange odor. Follow your nose and eyes—even if the expiration date is OK, pass on any fresh food that has a strange smell or that looks unusual.

- Place meats in plastic bags so that any juices do not leak onto other foods in your cart.

- Ground beef should be red, not any shade of brown.

- Eyeball eggs before buying them. Make sure that none of the eggs are cracked and that they are all clean. Eggs should be grade A or AA.

✎ Weird Words

Escherichia Coli (E. coli): Bacteria that cause infection and irritation of the large intestine. The bacteria are spread by unclean water, dirty cooking utensils, or undercooked meat.

Campylobacter: A type of bacteria associated with foodborne illness characterized by diarrhea, abdominal pain, fever, and vomiting.

Foodborne Illness: An acute gastrointestinal infection caused by food that contains harmful bacteria. Symptoms include diarrhea, abdominal pain, fever, and chills; also called food poisoning.

Salmonellosis: A type of foodborne illness caused by the bacterium _Salmonella_; it may cause intestinal infection and diarrhea.

Don't slow down your cart for these bad-news foods:

- fruit with broken skin (bacteria can enter through the skin and contaminate the fruit)

- unpasteurized ciders or juices (they can contain harmful bacteria)

- prestuffed turkeys or chickens

In The Kitchen

After a trip to the market, the first things you should put away are those that belong in the refrigerator and freezer. Keep eggs in the original carton on a shelf in the fridge (most refrigerator doors don't keep eggs cold enough).

Ready to cook but not sure how quickly things should be used, how long they should cook, or what should be washed? Here are some important guidelines:

- Raw meat, poultry, or fish should be cooked or frozen within 2 days.

- Thaw frozen meat, poultry, and fish in the refrigerator or microwave, never at room temperature.

- Cook thawed meat, poultry, and fish immediately—don't let it hang around for hours.

- Cook meat until the center is no longer pink and the juices run clear.

- Cook crumbled ground beef or poultry until it's no longer pink.

> ### ♣ It's A Fact!!
>
> - Raw or undercooked eggs and poultry products can transmit *Salmonella* and cause illness.
>
> - Undercooked hamburger can transmit *E. coli*.

- Scrub all fruits and veggies with plain water to remove any leftover pesticides or dirt.

- Remove the outer leaves of leafy greens, such as spinach or lettuce.

- Don't let eggs hang out at room temperature for more than 2 hours.

- Make sure that you cook eggs thoroughly—no runny stuff.

Clean Up

Even though the kitchen might look clean, your hands, the countertops, and the utensils you use could still contain lots of bacteria that you can't even see. Yuck! To prevent the spread of bacteria while you're preparing food, check out the following:

- Always wash your hands with hot water and soap before preparing any food.

- Wash your hands after handling raw meat, poultry, fish, or egg products.

- Keep raw meats and their juices away from other foods in the refrigerator and on countertops.

- Never put cooked food on a dish that was holding raw meat, poultry, or fish.

- If you use knives and other utensils on raw meat, poultry, or fish, you need to wash them before using them to cut or handle something else.

- If you touch raw meat, poultry, or fish, wash your hands. Don't wipe them on a dishtowel—this can contaminate the towel with bacteria, which may be spread to someone else's hands.

- Use one cutting board for raw meat, poultry, and fish, and another board for everything else.

- When you're done preparing food, it's a good idea to wipe down the countertops with a commercial cleaning product. Don't forget to wash the cutting board in hot, soapy water and then disinfect it with a commercial cleaning product. You can also mix together 1 teaspoon chlorine bleach and 1 quart of water for a homemade cleaning solution and store the solution in a spray bottle. Of course, keep the solution and the ingredients out of the reach of your younger brothers and sisters!

Storing Leftovers Safely

Yum! Your dinner was a success and you're lucky to have some left over. Make sure you know the lowdown on leftovers:

- Put leftovers in the fridge as soon as possible. If you leave leftovers out for too long at room temperature, bacteria can quickly multiply, turning your delightful dish into a food poisoning disaster.

- Store leftovers in containers with lids that can be snapped tightly shut. Bowls or tins are OK for storing leftovers, but be sure to cover them tightly with plastic wrap or aluminum foil to keep the food from drying out.

- Eat any leftovers within 3 to 5 days or freeze them. Don't freeze any dishes that contain uncooked fruit or veggies, hard-cooked eggs, or mayonnaise.

- If you're freezing leftovers, freeze them in one- or two-portion servings, so they'll be easy to take out of the freezer, pop in the microwave, and eat.

- Store leftovers in plastic containers, plastic bags, or aluminum foil. Don't fill bowls all the way to the top; when food is frozen, it expands. Leave a little extra space—about 1/2 inch should do it.

- Eat frozen leftovers within 2 months.

> ♣ **It's A Fact!!**
>
> Because most refrigerator doors don't keep eggs cold enough, eggs should be kept in the original carton on a shelf inside the fridge.

Microwave Magic

It's easy to make magic with your microwave—you can heat up or defrost stuff in an instant. Before touching that power button, be sure you know what you can microwave and how to do it:

- Use only utensils and containers that are approved for use in the microwave.

- Although plastic plates and bowls are usually OK for use in the microwave, don't use margarine tubs or cottage cheese containers. The heat can melt them, which means that some of the chemicals in the plastic can be transferred into your food.

- Most glass and ceramic containers are OK for use in the microwave. If you're not sure about glass, here's an easy test: microwave the empty container for 1 minute. If you remove it and the glass is cool, it's OK for cooking. If the glass is warm, it's unsafe.

- Waxed paper is safe for use in the microwave, but don't ever use brown paper or brown grocery bags. And never use aluminum foil!

- When covering a plate or container with plastic wrap, try to keep the plastic wrap from touching the food.

- If a food comes packaged in a foam tray, remove it from the tray and be sure to take off any plastic wrapping before microwaving. The heat can make foam trays and plastic wrapping melt. And don't reuse trays that are included with microwave dinners or other foods.

- If you're using the microwave to defrost foods, finish cooking them right away.

- If you're using the microwave to cook foods, be sure to move the food inside the dish or stir it several times so it cooks thoroughly.

- If you're using the microwave to heat leftovers or frozen meals, the food should be very hot to the touch and steaming.

- Always carefully follow the microwave directions on the box, especially the length of cooking time that's specified.

☞ Remember!!

Food safety concerns revolve around three main functions: food storage, food handling, and cooking. Taking the time to follow a few common-sense procedures can help ensure that you and the people you serve stay healthy.

Part Four
Weight Control

Chapter 28

Should You Go On A Diet?

What do the hula hoop, "high-protein diets," and wearing your clothes backwards have in common? They are all fads. Fads come and go, but when it comes to fad diets, the health effects can be permanent—especially for teenagers.

Not all teens who go on diets need to lose weight. Pressure from friends—and sometimes parents—to be very slim may create a distorted body image. Having a distorted body image is like looking into a funhouse mirror: You see yourself as fatter than you are.

A national survey of 11,631 high school students conducted by the national Centers for Disease Control and Prevention found that more than a third of the girls considered themselves overweight, compared with fewer than 15 percent of the boys. More than 43 percent of the girls reported that they were on a diet—and a quarter of these dieters didn't think they were overweight. The survey found that the most common dieting methods used were skipping meals, taking diet pills, and inducing vomiting after eating.

"The teenage years are a period of rapid growth and development," points out Ronald Kleinman, M.D., chief of the Pediatric Gastrointestinal and Nutrition Unit of Massachusetts General Hospital in Boston. He explains

About This Chapter: The text in this chapter is from article by Ruth Papazian that originally appeared in the September 1993 *FDA Consumer*. This version is from a reprint of that article, Publication No. (FDA) 97-1214; it contains revisions made in May 1994 and May 1997.

that fad dieting can keep teenagers from getting the calories and nutrients they need to grow properly and that dieting can retard growth. Stringent dieting may cause girls to stop menstruating, and will prevent boys from developing muscles, he says. If the diet doesn't provide enough calcium, phosphorus, and vitamin D, bones may not lay down enough calcium. This may increase the risk of osteoporosis later in life, although more studies are needed to confirm this.

Instead of dieting because "everyone" is doing it or because you are not as thin as you want to be, first find out from a doctor or nutritionist whether you are carrying too much body fat for your age and height.

What If You Need To Lose Weight?

The flip side to feeling pressured to be thin is having legitimate concerns about overweight that adults dismiss by saying, "It's just baby fat" or "You'll grow into your weight." Most girls reach almost their full height once they start to menstruate, notes Kleinman. Although boys usually don't stop growing until age 18, data from a study suggest that adolescent obesity can carry serious lifelong health consequences for them.

The study, which followed the medical histories of 508 people from childhood to age 70, found that men who had been overweight teenagers were more likely to develop colon cancer and to suffer fatal heart attacks and strokes than their thinner classmates. Women who had been overweight teens had an increased tendency to develop clogged arteries (atherosclerosis) and arthritis. By age 70, these problems made it difficult for them to walk more than a quarter mile, lift heavy objects, or climb stairs.

While this study linked adolescent obesity to health problems decades down the road, some adverse effects show up much earlier. Sometimes teens develop high blood pressure, elevated cholesterol, and conditions that often precede diabetes. Also, as Kleinman points out, "The longer in adolescence you remain overweight, the greater the likelihood that the problem will persist into adulthood."

As with most everything else, there's a right way and a wrong way to lose weight. The wrong way is to skip meals, resolve to eat nothing but diet bread and water, take diet pills, or make yourself vomit. You may make it through the end of the week and maybe even lose a pound or two, but you're unlikely to keep the weight off for more than a few months—if that. And inducing vomiting can lead to an eating disorder called bulimia, which can result in serious health problems.

"The more you deprive yourself of the foods you love, the more you will crave those foods. Inevitably, you'll break down and binge," says Jo Ann Hattner, a clinical dietitian at Packard Children's Hospital in Palo Alto, California. Then you'll not only gain those pounds back, you'll likely add a couple more.

Experts call this cycle of weight loss and weight gain "yo-yo" dieting. Obesity researchers believe that truly overweight people should continue to try to control their weight because studies are inconclusive on whether weight cycling is harmful, according to the National Institute of Diabetes and Digestive and Kidney Diseases. In contrast, the health risks from being overweight are well-known. Although the yo-yo effect may not hurt future weight-loss efforts, you need to make lifelong changes in eating behavior, diet, and physical activity.

Additionally, low-calorie diets that allow only a few types of foods can be bad for your health because they don't allow you to get enough vitamins and minerals. Kleinman warns that rapid weight loss from very low-calorie "starvation diets" can cause serious effects in teenagers, such as gallstones, hair loss, weakness, and diarrhea.

Diet Pills

In 1992, FDA banned 111 ingredients in over-the-counter (OTC) diet products—including amino acids, cellulose, and grapefruit extract—after manufacturers were unable to prove that they worked.

A number of products (Cal-Ban 3000, Cal-Lite 1000, Cal-Trim 5000, Perma Slim, Bodi Trim, Dictol 7 Plus, Medi Thin, Nature's Way, and East Indian Guar Gum) were also recalled because they posed serious health risks. The products contained guar gum, which supposedly swelled in the stomach to provide a feeling of fullness. However, the swelling from the guar gum caused blockages in the throat and stomach.

In February 1996, FDA also proposed new warning labels for OTC diet pills containing phenylpropanolamine (PPA), including the statement that the product is "For use by people 18 years of age and older."

PPA is an ingredient found not only in many OTC diet pills but also in cough-cold and allergy products as well. FDA is concerned PPA may possibly increase the risk of a type of stroke (hemorrhagic) caused by bleeding into the brain, as was suggested by some reports of bleeding in the brain among PPA users, typically young women. This possible risk could be further increased if a person took more than the recommended dose of PPA, which might occur inadvertently from also taking a cough-cold product with PPA.

While FDA agrees that studies have not shown a definite link between PPA and stroke, the agency believes data from a more comprehensive study are needed to confirm the ingredient's safety. As a result, the OTC drug industry began a five-year study in 1994.

Michael Weintraub, M.D, director of FDA's Office of Drug Evaluation V, says, "PPA is not recommended for use by teenagers also because they are still growing and if they suppress their appetite, they may not get proper nutrition." The author of studies on PPA published in scientific journals, Weintraub adds, "This is especially true of teens who don't need to lose weight but think that they do."

The Real Skinny On Weight Loss

If going to extremes won't do the trick, what will? Believe it or not, it's as simple as making a few changes in your eating habits to emphasize healthy foods and exercise—good advice even if you don't need to lose weight.

> ✤ It's A Fact!!
>
> Low-calorie diets that allow only a few types of foods can be bad for your health because they don't allow you to get enough vitamins and minerals. Fad or starvation diets and diet pills offer temporary solutions, at best. At worst, they may jeopardize your health.

✔ Quick Tip

The WRONG way to lose weight:

- skip meals
- eat only bread and water
- take diet pills
- induce vomiting

The RIGHT way to lose weight:

- eat healthy foods
- exercise at least three time a week

Hattner describes a good diet as one that has balance, variety and moderation in food choices. She suggests using the U.S. Department of Agriculture's "Food Pyramid." These guidelines call for six to 11 servings a day of grains (bread, cereal, rice and pasta), three to five servings of vegetables, two to four servings of fruit, and two to three servings each of dairy (milk, cheese and yogurt) and protein-rich foods (meat, eggs, poultry, fish, dry beans, and nuts).

"The most important dietary change you can make is to limit the amount of high-fat foods that you eat," she adds. "Balance your favorite foods [which are usually high in fat] with fruits and vegetables [which are almost always very low in fat]; eat a wide variety of foods to keep from getting bored and to make sure your diet is nutritionally sound; and keep portion sizes reasonable so that you can have your [thin] slice of cake and lose weight, too."

To keep fat intake down, Hattner recommends making simple lower fat substitutions for the foods that you eat: Switch to 1 percent or skim milk instead of whole milk, nonfat or low-fat frozen yogurt or nonfat or low-fat ice cream instead of regular ice cream, and pretzels instead of corn chips. High-fat foods such as french fries, candy bars, and milkshakes that have no low-fat substitutes should only be eaten once in a while or in very small amounts.

Move It And Lose It

Whether you are overweight or not, regular exercise (at least three times a week) is important to look and feel your best. If you do need to lose weight, stepping up your activity level will cause you to burn calories more quickly and help make weight loss easier.

"Exercise increases lean body weight. Also, you will appear slimmer as you develop your muscles because muscles give shape and form to your body," notes Hattner.

Fad or starvation diets and diet pills offer temporary solutions, at best. At worst, they may jeopardize your health. According to Weintraub, "The safest way for teenagers to control their weight is to eat a healthy, low-fat diet and get enough exercise."

☞ Remember!!

A healthy diet is one that has balance, variety, and moderation in food choices.

Chapter 29

Overweight: A Weight Reduction Program For Teenagers

Description

- You appear overweight.

- You weigh more than 20 percent over the ideal weight for your height.

- The skin fold thickness of your upper arm's fat layer is more than 1 inch (25 millimeters) when measured with a special instrument.

  More than 25 percent of American teenagers are overweight.

Causes

The tendency to be overweight is usually inherited. If one parent is overweight, probably half of the children will be overweight. If both parents are overweight, most of their children will be overweight. If neither parent is overweight, the children have a 10 percent chance of being overweight.

Heredity alone (without overeating) accounts for most mild obesity, whereas moderate obesity is usually due to a combination of heredity, overeating, and underexercising. Some overeating is normal in our society, but

About This Chapter: Text in this chapter is from "Overweight: A Weight Reduction Program (for Teenagers)," by B.D. Schmitt in *Clinical Reference Systems*, July 1, 1999 p1098, © 1999 Clinical Reference Systems; reprinted with permission.

only those who have the inherited tendency to be overweight will gain significant weight when they overeat.

Less than 1 percent of obesity has an underlying medical cause. Your physician can easily determine whether your obesity has a physical cause with a simple physical examination.

> ✎ **Weird Words**
>
> Skin Fold Thickness: A measurement taken using special calipers to estimate the amount of fat under the skin.

Expected Course

Losing weight is very difficult. Keeping the weight off is also a chore. The best time for losing weight is when a teenager becomes very concerned with personal appearance. A self-motivated teenager can follow a diet and lose weight regardless of what his or her family eats.

How To Lose Weight

Motivation

You can increase your motivation by joining a weight-loss club such as TOPS or Weight Watchers. Sometimes schools have classes for helping teenagers lose weight.

Setting Weight-Loss Goals

Pick a realistic target weight dependent on your bone structure and degree of obesity. The loss of 1 pound a week is an attainable goal. However, you will have to work quite hard to lose this much weight every week for several weeks. You should weigh yourself no more than once each week; daily weighings generate too much false hope or disappointment. When losing weight becomes a strain, take a few weeks off from the weight-loss program. During this time, try to stay at a constant weight.

Once you have reached the target weight, the long-range goal is to try to stay within 5 pounds of that weight. Staying at a particular weight is possible only through a permanent moderation in eating. You will probably always have the tendency to gain weight easily and it's important that you understand this.

Diet: Decreasing Calorie Consumption

You should eat three well-balanced meals a day of average-sized portions. There are no forbidden foods; you can have a serving of anything family or friends are eating. However, there are forbidden portions. While you are reducing, you must leave the table a bit hungry. You cannot lose weight if you eat until full (satiated). Eat average portions instead of large portions and avoid seconds. Shortcuts such as fasting, crash dieting, or diet pills rarely work and may be dangerous. Liquid diets are safe only if they are used according to directions.

Calorie counting is helpful for some people, but it is usually too time-consuming. Consider the following guidelines on what to eat and drink:

- *Fluids:* Mainly drink low-calorie drinks such as skim milk, fruit juice diluted in half with water, diet drinks, or flavored mineral water. Because milk has lots of calories, drink no more than 16 ounces of skim, 1-percent, or 2-percent milk each day. Drink no more than 8 ounces of fruit juice a day. All other drinks should be either water or diet drinks. Try to drink six glasses of water each day.

- *Meals:* Eat fewer fatty foods (for example, eggs, bacon, sausage, and butter). A portion of fat has twice as many calories as the same portion of protein or carbohydrate. Trim the fat off meats. Eat more baked, broiled, boiled, or steamed foods and fewer fried foods. Eat more fruits, vegetables, salads, and grains.

- *Desserts:* Try to eat smaller-than-average portions of desserts. Try more Jell-O and fresh fruits as desserts. Avoid rich desserts. Do not eat second helpings.

- *Snacks:* Eat mainly low-calorie foods such as raw vegetables (carrot sticks, celery sticks, raw potato sticks, pickles, etc.), raw fruits (apples, oranges, cantaloupe, etc.), popcorn, or diet soft drinks. You should have no more than two snacks a day.

- *Vitamins:* Take one multivitamin tablet daily during your weight-loss program.

Eating Habits

To counteract the tendency to gain weight, you must learn eating habits that will last you for a lifetime.

- Don't skip any of the three basic meals.

- Drink a glass of water before meals.

- Eat smaller portions.

- Chew your food slowly.

- Avoid high-calorie snack foods such as potato chips, candy, or regular soft drinks.

- Do keep available diet soft drinks, fresh fruits, and vegetables.

> ✔ **Quick Tip**
>
> Avoid the temptation to weigh yourself frequently. Daily weighings generate too much false hope or disappointment. A better plan is to weigh yourself no more than once a week.

- Leave only low-calorie snacks out on the counter—fruit, for example. Put away the cookie jar.

- Store food only in the kitchen. Keep it out of other rooms.

- Eat no more than two snacks each day. Avoid continual snacking ("grazing") throughout the day.

- Eat only at the kitchen or dining-room table. Don't eat while watching TV, studying, riding in a car, or shopping in a store. Once eating becomes associated with these activities, the body learns to expect it.

- Don't eat alone.

- Reward yourself for hard work or studying with a movie, TV, music, or a book instead of food.

- Post some reminder cards on the refrigerator and bathroom mirror that state "EAT LESS" or "STICK TO THE PROGRAM."

Exercise: Increasing Calorie Expenditure

Daily exercise can increase the rate of weight loss as well as the sense of physical well-being. The combination of diet and exercise is the most effective way to lose weight. Try the following forms of exercise:

- Walking or riding a bicycle instead of riding in a car.

- Using stairs instead of elevators.

- Learning new sports. Swimming and jogging are the sports that burn the most calories. Your school may have an aerobics class.

- Taking the dog for a long walk.

- Spending 30 minutes a day exercising or dancing to records or music on TV.

- Using an exercise bike or Hula Hoop while watching TV. (Limit your TV sitting time to 2 hours or less each day.)

Social Activities: Keeping The Mind Off Food

The more outside activities you participate in, the easier it will be for you to lose weight. Spare time fosters nibbling. Most snacking occurs between 3 and 6 p.m. Fill after-school time with activities such as music, drama, sports, or scouts. A part-time job after school may help. If nothing else, call or visit friends. An active social life almost always leads to weight reduction.

When To Call Your Doctor

Call your physician during office hours if:

- You have not improved your eating and exercise habits after trying this program for 2 months.

- You are a compulsive overeater.

- You are depressed.

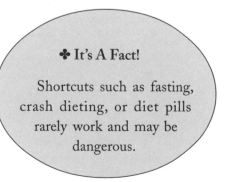

❖ **It's A Fact!**

Shortcuts such as fasting, crash dieting, or diet pills rarely work and may be dangerous.

- You feel you have no close friends.

- You have other questions or concerns.

☞ **Remember!!**

Not all teens who go on diets need to lose weight. But if you have legitimate concerns about being overweight—for example, if you weigh more than 20 percent over the ideal weight for your height—a weight loss program may be the right choice for you.

Although losing weight is difficult and keeping the weight off is also a chore, a combination of a healthy diet and regular exercise is an effective way to control weight.

Chapter 30

Weight Loss For Life

How We Lose Weight

Your body weight is controlled by the number of calories you eat and the number of calories you use each day. So, to lose weight you need to take in fewer calories than you use. You can do this by becoming more physically active or by eating less. Following a weight-loss program that helps you to become more physically active and decrease the amount of calories that you eat is most likely to lead to successful weight loss. The weight-loss program should also help you keep the weight off by making changes in your physical activity and eating habits that you will be able to follow for the rest of your life.

Types Of Weight-Loss Programs

To lose weight and keep it off, you should be aware of the different types of programs available and the important parts of a good program. Knowing this information should help you select or design a weight-loss program that will work for you. The three types of weight-loss programs include: do-it-yourself programs, non-clinical programs, and clinical programs.

About This Chapter: The text in this chapter is from "Weight Loss for Life," a pamphlet by the National Institute of Diabetes and Digestive and Kidney Diseases (NIDDK), January 1998.

Do-It-Yourself Programs

Any effort to lose weight by yourself or with a group of like-minded others through support groups, worksite or community-based programs fits in the "do-it yourself" category. Individuals using a do-it-yourself program rely on their own judgment, group support, and products such as diet books for advice (Note: Not all diet books are reliable sources of weight-loss information).

✎ Weird Words

Bariatrician: A doctor specializing in obesity prevention and treatment.

Counselor: A person who provides guidance; licensing requirements vary according to state law.

Registered Dietician: A professional who provides nutrition care services and dietary counseling for both healthy and sick individuals. A registered dietician (RD) must complete a bachelor's or a graduate degree with a program in dietetics/nutrition and complete an approved program in dietetic practice such as an internship.

Nurse: A professional who provides health care services, often under the direction of a doctor. Different types of nurses have varying amounts of education and professional experience. A licensed practical nurse (L.P.N) has 12 to 18 months of training. A registered nurse (RN) may have 2, 3, or 4 years of education in a nursing school. A nurse practitioner (NP) has training beyond basic nursing.

Nutritionist: A title used by a wide range of people, including registered dietitians but also including people who have taken correspondence or other short-term courses in nutrition and even people who are self-taught. Before seeking the advice of a health practitioner in nutrition, it is a good idea to ask what kind of training and practical experience the person has received.

Psychologist: A health professional trained and licensed to assess, diagnose, and treat people with mental, emotional, or behavioral disorders.

Non-Clinical Programs

These programs may or may not be commercially operated, such as through a privately-owned, weight-loss chain. They often use books and pamphlets that are prepared by health-care providers. These programs use counselors (who usually are not health-care providers and may or may not have training) to provide services to you. Some programs require participants to use the program's food or supplements.

Clinical Programs

This type of program may or may not be commercially owned. Services are provided in a health-care setting, such as a hospital, by licensed health professionals, such as physicians, nurses, dietitians, and/or psychologists. In some clinical programs, a health professional works alone; in others, a group of health professionals works together to provide services to patients. Clinical programs may offer you services such as nutrition education, medical care, behavior change therapy, and physical activity.

Clinical programs may also use other weight-loss methods, such as very low-calorie diets, prescription weight-loss drugs, and surgery, to treat severely overweight patients. These treatments are described below:

Very low-calorie diets (VLCDs) are commercially prepared formulas that provide no more than 800 calories per day and replace all usual food intake. VLCDs help individuals lose weight more quickly than is usually possible with low-calorie diets. Because VLCDs can cause side effects, obesity experts recommend that only people who are severely overweight use these diets, and only with proper medical care. A fact sheet on VLCDs is available from the Weight-control Information Network (WIN).

Prescribed weight-loss drugs should be used only if you are likely to have health problems caused by your weight. You should not use drugs to improve your appearance. Prescribed weight-loss drugs, when combined with a healthy diet and regular physical activity, may help some obese adults lose weight. However, before these medications can be widely recommended, more research is needed to determine their long-term safety and effectiveness. Whatever the results, prescription weight-loss drugs should be used only as part of an overall program that includes long-term changes in your eating and physical activity habits. A fact sheet on prescription medications for the treatment of obesity is available from WIN.

You may consider **gastric surgery** to promote weight loss if you are more than 80 pounds overweight. The surgery, sometimes called bariatric surgery, causes weight loss in one of two ways: 1) by limiting the amount of food your stomach can hold by closing off or removing parts of the stomach or 2) by causing food to be poorly digested by bypassing the stomach or part of the intestines. After surgery, patients usually lose weight quickly. While some weight is often regained, many patients are successful in keeping off most of their weight. In some cases, the surgery can lead to problems that require follow-up operations. Surgery may also reduce the amount of vitamins and minerals in your body and cause gallstones. For additional information, a fact sheet on gastric surgery is available from WIN.

If you are considering a weight-loss program and you have medical problems, or if you are severely overweight, programs run by trained health professionals may be best for you. These professionals are more likely to monitor you for possible side effects of weight loss and to talk to your doctor when necessary.

> **✔ Quick Tip**
> Whether you decide to use the do-it-yourself, non-clinical, or clinical approach, the program should help you lose weight and keep it off by teaching you healthy eating and physical activity habits that you will be able to follow for the rest of your life.

Diet

The word "diet" probably brings to mind meals of lettuce and cottage cheese. By definition, "diet" refers to what a person eats or drinks during the course of a day. A diet that limits portions to a very small size or that excludes certain foods entirely to promote weight loss may not be effective over the long term. Rather, you are likely to miss certain foods and find it difficult to follow this type of diet for a long time. Instead, it is often helpful to gradually change the types and amounts of food you eat and maintain these changes for the rest of your life. The ideal diet is one that takes into account your likes and dislikes and includes a wide variety of foods with enough calories and nutrients for good health.

How much you eat and what you eat play a major role in how much you weigh. So, when planning your diet, you should consider: What calorie level is appropriate? Is the diet you are considering nutritionally balanced? Will the diet be practical and easy to follow? Will you be able to maintain this eating plan for the rest of your life? The following information will help you answer these questions.

Low-Calorie Diets

Most weight-loss diets provide 1,000 to 1,500 calories per day. However, the number of calories that is right for you depends on your weight and activity level. At these calorie levels, diets are referred to as low-calorie diets. Self-help diet books and clinical and non-clinical weight-loss programs often include low-calorie diet plans.

The calorie level of your diet should allow for a weight loss of no more than 1 pound per week (after the first week or two when weight loss may be more rapid because of initial water loss). If you can estimate how many calories you eat in a day, you can design a diet plan that will help you lose no more than 1 pound per week. You may need to work with a trained health professional, such as a registered dietitian. Or, you can use a standardized low-calorie diet plan with a fixed calorie level. The selected calorie level, however, may not produce the recommended rate of weight loss, and you may need to eat more or less.

Good Nutrition

Make sure that your diet contains all the essential nutrients for good health. Using the Food Guide Pyramid (see Chapter 12) and the Nutrition Facts Label that is found on most processed food products can help you choose a healthful diet. The Pyramid shows you the kinds and amounts of food that you need each day for good health. The Nutrition Facts Label will help you select foods that meet your daily nutritional needs. A healthful diet should include:

Adequate vitamins and minerals. Eating a wide variety of foods from all the food groups on the Food Guide Pyramid will help you get the vitamins and minerals you need. If you eat less than 1,200 calories per day, you may benefit from taking a daily vitamin and mineral supplement.

Adequate protein. The average woman 25 years of age and older should get 50 grams of protein each day, and the average man 25 years of age and older should get 63 grams of protein each day. Adequate protein is important because it prevents muscle tissue from breaking down and repairs all body tissues such as skin and teeth. To get adequate protein in your diet, make sure you eat 2-3 servings from the Meat, Poultry, Fish, Dry Beans, Eggs, and Nuts Group on the Food Guide Pyramid every day. These foods are all good sources of protein.

Adequate carbohydrates. At least 100 grams of carbohydrates per day are needed to prevent fatigue and dangerous fluid imbalances. To make sure you get enough carbohydrates, eat 6-11 servings from the Bread, Cereal, Rice, and Pasta Group on the Food Guide Pyramid every day.

A daily fiber intake of 20 to 30 grams. Adequate fiber helps with proper bowel function. If you were to eat 1 cup of bran cereal, 1/2 cup of carrots, 1/2 cup of kidney beans, a medium-sized pear, and a medium-sized apple together in 1 day, you would get about 30 grams of fiber.

No more than 30 percent of calories, on average, from fat per day, with less than 10 percent of calories from saturated fat (such as fat from meat, butter, and eggs). Limiting fat to these levels reduces your risk for heart disease and may help you lose weight. In addition, you should limit the amount of cholesterol in your diet. Cholesterol is a fat-like substance found in animal products such as meat and eggs. Your diet should include no more than 300 milligrams of cholesterol per day (one egg contains about 215 milligrams of cholesterol, and 3.5 ounces of cooked hamburger contain 100 milligrams of cholesterol).

At least 8 to 10 glasses, 8 ounces each, of water or water-based beverages, per day. You need more water if you exercise a lot.

These nutrients should come from a variety of low-calorie, nutrient-rich foods. One way to get variety—and with it, an enjoyable and nutritious diet—is to choose foods each day from the Food Guide Pyramid.

Types Of Diets

Fixed-menu diet. A fixed-menu diet provides a list of all the foods you will eat. This kind of diet can be easy to follow because the foods are selected for you. But, you get very few different food choices which may make the diet boring and hard to follow away from home. In addition, fixed-menu diets do not teach the food selection skills necessary for keeping weight off. If you start with a fixed-menu diet, you should switch eventually to a plan that helps you learn to make meal choices on your own, such as an exchange-type diet.

Exchange-type diet. An exchange-type diet is a meal plan with a set number of servings from each of several food groups. Within each group, foods are about equal in calories and can be interchanged as you wish. For example, the "starch" category could include one slice of bread or 1/2 cup of oatmeal; each is about equal in nutritional value and calories. If your meal plan calls for two starch choices at breakfast, you could choose to eat two slices of bread, or one slice of bread and 1/2 cup of oatmeal. With the exchange-type diet plans, you have more day-to-day variety and you can easily follow the diet away from home. The most important advantage is that exchange-type diet plans teach the food selection skills you need to keep your weight off.

Prepackaged-meal diet. These diets require you to buy prepackaged meals. Such meals may help you learn appropriate portion sizes. However, they can be costly. Before beginning this type of program, find out whether you will need to buy the meals and how much the meals cost. You should also find out whether the program will teach you how to select and prepare food, skills that are needed to sustain weight loss.

Formula diet. Formula diets are weight-loss plans that replace one or more meals with a liquid formula. Most formula diets are balanced diets containing a mix of protein, carbohydrate, and usually a small amount of fat. Formula diets are usually sold as liquid or a powder to be mixed with liquid. Although formula diets are easy to use and do promote short-term weight loss, most people regain the weight as soon as they stop using the formula. In addition, formula diets do not teach you how to make healthy food choices, a necessary skill for keeping your weight off.

Questionable diets. You should avoid any diet that suggests you eat a certain nutrient, food, or combination of foods to promote easy weight loss. Some of these diets may work in the short term because they are low in calories. However, they are often not well balanced and may cause nutrient deficiencies. In addition, they do not teach eating habits that are important for long-term weight management.

Flexible diets. Some programs or books suggest monitoring fat only, calories only, or a combination of the two, with the individual making the choice of both the type and amount of food eaten. This flexible type of approach works well for many people, and teaches them how to control what they eat. One drawback of flexible diets is that some don't consider the total diet. For example, programs that monitor fat only often allow people to take in unlimited amounts of excess calories from sugars, and therefore don't lead to weight loss.

It is important to choose an eating plan that you can live with. The plan should also teach you how to select and prepare healthy foods, as well as how to maintain your new weight. Remember that many people tend to regain lost weight. Eating a healthful and nutritious diet to maintain your new weight, combined with regular physical activity, helps to prevent weight regain.

Physical Activity

Regular physical activity is important to help you lose weight and build an overall healthy lifestyle. Physical activity increases the number of calories your body uses and promotes the loss of body fat instead of muscle and other nonfat tissue. Research shows that people who include physical activity in their weight-loss programs are more likely to keep their weight off than people who only change their diet. In addition to promoting weight control, physical activity improves your strength and flexibility, lowers your risk of heart disease, helps control blood pressure and diabetes, can promote a sense of well-being, and can decrease stress.

Any type of physical activity you choose to do—vigorous activities such as running or aerobic dancing or moderate-intensity activities such as walking or household work—will increase the number of calories your body uses. The key to successful weight control and improved overall health is making physical activity a part of your daily life.

For the greatest overall health benefits, experts recommend that you do 20 to 30 minutes of vigorous physical activity three or more times a week and some type of muscle strengthening activity, such as weight resistance, and stretching at least twice a week. However, if you are unable to do this level of activity, you can improve your health by performing 30 minutes or more of moderate-intensity physical activity over the course of a day, at least five times a week. When including physical activity in your weight-loss program, you should choose a variety of activities that can be done regularly and are enjoyable for you. Also, if you have not been physically active, you should see your doctor before you start, especially if you are older than 40 years of age, very overweight, or have medical problems. A fact sheet on physical activity and weight control is available from WIN.

Moderate-Intensity Activities

- walking up the stairs instead of taking the elevator

- walking part or all of the way to work

- using a push mower to cut the grass

- playing actively with children

Vigorous Activities

- aerobic dancing
- running
- brisk walking
- cycling
- swimming

Behavior Change

Behavior change focuses on learning eating and physical activity behaviors that will help you lose weight and keep it off. The first step is to look at your eating and physical activity habits, thus uncovering behaviors (such as television watching) that lead you to overeat or be inactive. Next you'll need to learn how to change those behaviors.

♣ It's A Fact!

You may find some of the following publications helpful sources of additional information:

"Binge Eating Disorder," NIH Publication No. 94-3589. This fact sheet describes the symptoms, causes, complications, and treatment of binge eating disorder, along with a profile of those at risk for the disorder. 1993. Available from WIN.

"Dieting and Gallstones," NIH Publication No. 94-3677. This fact sheet describes what gallstones are, how weight loss may cause them, and how to lessen the risk of developing them. 1993. Available from WIN.

"Gastric Surgery for Severe Obesity," NIH Publication No. 96-4006. This fact sheet describes the different types of surgery available to treat severe obesity. It explains how gastric surgery promotes weight loss and the benefits and risks of each procedure. 1996. Available from WIN.

"Physical Activity and Weight Control," NIH Publication No. 96-4031. This fact sheet explains how physical activity helps promote weight control and other ways it benefits one's health. It also describes the different types of physical activity and provides tips on how to become more physically active. 1996. Available from WIN.

"Prescription Medications for the Treatment of Obesity," NIH Publication No. 97-4191. This fact sheet presents information on appetite suppressant medications. These medications may help some obese patients lose more weight than with non-drug treatments. The types of medications and the risks and benefits associated with the use of these medications are described. Revised 1997. Available from WIN.

"Very Low-Calorie Diets," NIH Publication No. 95-3894. Information on who should use a very low-calorie diet (VLCD) and the health benefits and possible adverse effects of VLCDs is provided in this fact sheet. 1995. Available from WIN.

"Weight Cycling," NIH Publication No. 95-3901. Based on research, this fact sheet describes the health effects of weight cycling, also known as "yo-yo" dieting, and how it affects obese individuals' future weight-loss efforts. 1995. Available from WIN.

Getting support from others is a good way to help you maintain your new eating and physical activity habits. Changing your eating and physical activity behaviors increases your chances of losing weight and keeping it off. For additional information on behavior change, you may wish to ask a weight-loss counselor or refer to books on this topic, which are available in local libraries.

"Are You Eating Right?" *Consumer Reports*. October 1992, pp. 644-55. This article summarizes advice from 68 nutrition experts, including a discussion on weight control and health risks of obesity. Available from WIN.

"Losing Weight: What Works. What Doesn't" and "Rating the Diets." *Consumer Reports*. June 1993, pp. 347-57. These articles report on a survey of readers' experiences with weight-loss diets, discuss research related to weight control, and outline pros and cons of different diet programs. Available in public libraries.

"The Facts About Weight-Loss Products and Programs." DHHS Publication No. (FDA) 92-1189. This pamphlet provides basic facts about the weight-loss industry and what the consumer should expect from a diet program and/or product. Available from the Food and Drug Administration, Office of Consumer Affairs, HFE-88, Rockville, MD 20857.

"Nutrition and Your Health: Dietary Guidelines for Americans, Fourth Edition." Home and Garden Bulletin No. 232. 1995. This booklet answers some of the basic questions about healthy eating and the link between poor nutrition and disease. It stresses the importance of a balanced diet and a healthy lifestyle. Available from WIN.

"A Report of the Surgeon General: Physical Activity and Health," 1996. Produced by the Centers for Disease Control and Prevention, this report compiles decades of research concerning physical activity and health. It addresses the nationwide health problems associated with physical inactivity and outlines the benefits of becoming more physically active. Available for $19.00 from the U.S. Government Printing Office, Superintendent of Documents, Washington, DC 20402; (202) 512-1800. Stock Number 017-023-00196-5.

What Works For YOU?

A variety of options exist to help you lose weight and keep it off. The key to successful weight loss is making changes in your eating and physical activity habits that you will be able to maintain for the rest of your life.

Weight-Control Information Network (WIN)

1 WIN Way
Bethesda, MD 20892-3665
1-800-946-8098
(202) 828-1025
Fax: (202) 828-1028
E-mail: WIN@info.niddk.nih.gov
Internet: http://www.niddk.nih.gov/health/nutrit/win.htm

The Weight-control Information Network (WIN) is a service of the National Institute of Diabetes and Digestive and Kidney Diseases, part of the National Institutes of Health, under the U.S. Public Health Service. Authorized by Congress (Public Law 103-43), WIN assembles and disseminates to health professionals and the general public information on weight control, obesity, and nutritional disorders. WIN responds to requests for information; develops, reviews, and distributes publications; and develops communication strategies to encourage individuals to achieve and maintain a healthy weight.

Publications produced by WIN are reviewed for scientific accuracy, content, and readability. Materials produced by other sources are also reviewed for scientific accuracy and are distributed, along with WIN publications, to answer requests.

☞ **Remember!**

Following a weight-loss program that helps you to become more physically active and decrease the amount of calories that you eat is most likely to lead to successful weight loss.

Chapter 31

The Skinny On Dieting

Dieting is close to a national pastime. An estimated 50 million Americans will go on diets this year, and while some will succeed in taking off weight, experts suggest that very few—perhaps five percent—will manage to keep all of it off in the long run.

Although some people try to exercise off their excess pounds or inches, dieting is the most common way to lose weight. Recent surveys indicate that many dieters—more than 80 percent of women and 75 percent of men—eat fewer calories in their efforts to shed a few pounds. Unfortunately, simply cutting calories doesn't work for long.

Meanwhile, every year, about 8 million Americans enroll in some kind of structured weight-loss program involving liquid diets, special diet regimens, or medical or other supervision. Yet weight loss experts caution against fad diets, which rarely have a permanent effect. And they recommend that very-low calorie diets be pursued only under medical supervision because of their risks. The Federal Trade Commission (FTC) also advises consumers to be skeptical of plans or products that promote easy or effortless long-term weight loss. They just don't work, according to the agency, which oversees the advertising and marketing of foods, non-prescription drugs, medical devices and health care services.

About This Chapter: Text in this chapter is from a pamphlet titled "The Skinny on Dieting" produced by the Federal Trade Commission, March 1997.

Spotting Questionable Claims

How can you tell the sizzle from the substance when it comes to claims about weight-loss programs and products? The FTC suggests a healthy portion of skepticism. Here are some claims made by advertisers in recent years—and the facts.

"LOSE WEIGHT WHILE YOU SLEEP."

Fact: Losing weight requires significant changes affecting what kind of food—and how much—you eat. Claims for diet products and programs that promise weight loss without sacrifice or effort are bogus.

"LOSE WEIGHT AND KEEP IT OFF FOR GOOD."

Fact: Weight loss maintenance requires permanent changes in how you eat and how much you exercise. Be skeptical about products that claim you will keep off any weight permanently or for a long time.

> ♣ **It's A Fact!**
>
> Experts estimate that only about five percent of the people who lose weight actually maintain their weight loss.

"JOHN DOE LOST 84 POUNDS IN SIX WEEKS."

Fact: Someone else's claim of weight loss success may have little or no relevance to your own chances of success. Don't be misled.

"LOSE ALL THE WEIGHT YOU CAN FOR JUST $99."

Fact: There may be hidden costs. For example, some programs do not publicize the fact that you must buy prepackaged meals from them at costs that exceed program fees. Before you sign up for any weight loss program, ask for all the costs. Get them in writing.

"LOSE 30 POUNDS IN JUST 30 DAYS."

Fact: As a rule, the faster you lose weight, the more likely you are to gain it back. In addition, fast weight loss may harm your health. Unless you have a medical reason, don't look for programs that promise quick weight loss.

"SCIENTIFIC BREAKTHROUGH ... MEDICAL MIRACLE."

Fact: To lose weight, you have to reduce your intake of calories and increase your physical activity. Be skeptical of extravagant claims.

The Real Story

The FTC agrees with many health experts who recommend a combination of diet modification and exercise as the most effective way to lose weight and keep it off—and a goal of losing about a pound a week. A modest reduction of 500 calories a day will achieve this goal, because a total reduction of 3,500 calories is necessary to lose one pound of fat.

If you want to lose the proverbial "few pounds," the FTC suggests revising what you eat, cutting your caloric intake, and adding exercise to your weekly routine. Merely reducing calories often makes dieters feel hungry because it cuts down on important vitamins and minerals. This can end up sabotaging your efforts. Revising the diet by replacing many of the calories from fats with calories from other food groups and exercising several times a week to increase the use of calories should keep most people feeling full, satisfied, and motivated to continue healthful eating habits. Many health experts recommend that adults limit their fat consumption to 25 percent of total caloric intake.

✔ Quick Tip

If you have complaints about a weight loss program or product, contact your state Attorney General, local consumer protection office, or Better Business Bureau. Or you may file a complaint with the Federal Trade Commission (FTC). Write to Correspondence Branch, FTC, Washington, DC 20580. Although the FTC does not intervene in individual cases, the information you provide may indicate a pattern of possible law violations that require Commission actions.

The FTC publishes several brochures for consumers who are interested in weight loss programs and products. Write for Best Sellers, Public Reference Branch, Room 130, 6th and Pennsylvania Avenue, NW, Washington, D.C. 20580 or call (202) 326-2222; TDD: (202) 326-2502.

☞ Remember!

How can you lower your fat intake and cut your calories without feeling hungry, sacrificing important nutrients, or losing money? The FTC has the following suggestions:

- Before beginning any weight loss program, check with your doctor. Some diet plans have been associated with health complications. Make sure your diet is well-balanced, and meets dietary guidelines set by experts in clinical nutrition. In cases where obesity results in life threatening complications, medical intervention may be necessary.

- Consider all the alternatives before deciding on a product or program, including non-profit support groups, counseling services, physician-supervised programs, and self-discipline. Choose the one that's best for your needs and your budget.

- Follow a nutritionally sound diet plan. These often are available from hospitals, clinics, national health organizations, insurance companies, and health maintenance organizations. Most libraries also stock a variety of books that include healthful meal plans and recipes.

- Remember that individual diet needs vary according to body size, health, and level of activity.

- Create a meal plan that incorporates your food preferences or modify an existing plan to fit your tastes. Be realistic: A low-fat diet doesn't mean swearing off fatty foods forever. It means eating them once in a while.

- Increase your physical activity gradually. Regular physical exercise can help reduce and control weight by burning up calories.

- Pill power cannot replace will power. Successful weight loss depends on a personal commitment to changing your eating habits and increasing your levels of physical exercise. There are no magic bullets.

Chapter 32

Dieter's Brews Can Make You Sick

A cup of hot herbal tea may feel soothing to the soul, but instead of soothing the body, some herbal teas can make you sick.

This is especially true with so-called dieter's teas, herbal teas containing senna, aloe, buckthorn, and other plant-derived laxatives that, when consumed in excessive amounts, can cause diarrhea, vomiting, nausea, stomach cramps, chronic constipation, fainting, and perhaps death.

In recent years, the U.S. Food and Drug Administration (FDA) has received "adverse event" reports, including the deaths of four young women, in which dieter's teas may have been a contributing factor.

As a result, FDA is advising consumers to follow package directions carefully when using dieter's teas and other dietary supplements containing senna, aloe, and other stimulant laxatives. Consumers should seek medical attention for persistent diarrhea, abdominal cramps, and other bowel problems to prevent more serious complications.

The agency may consider requiring manufacturers to place a warning about the products' potential side effects on the products' labels. Some manufacturers already are doing so voluntarily.

About This Chapter: The text in this chapter is from " Dieter's Brews Make Tea Time A Dangerous Affair," by Paula Kurtzweil. This article originally appeared in the July-August 1997 *FDA Consumer*. The version reprinted here is from Publication No. (FDA) 97-1286, and it contains revisions made in December 1997.

These products—bought in health food stores and through mail-order catalogs, for example—often are used for weight loss based on some consumers' belief that increased bowel movements will prevent absorption of calories, thus preventing weight gain. However, a special committee of FDA's Food Advisory Committee concluded in 1995 that studies show that laxative-induced diarrhea does not significantly reduce absorption of calories. This is because the laxatives do not work on the small intestine, where calories are absorbed, but rather on the colon, the lower end of the bowel.

Juice drinks and tablets also may contain stimulant laxatives. FDA usually regulates these products as foods under the Federal Food, Drug, and Cosmetic Act. If the products are represented as dietary supplements, they are regulated under the Dietary Supplement Health and Education Act of 1994.

Stimulant Laxatives

The stimulant laxative teas and dietary supplements FDA is most concerned about contain one or more of the substances senna, aloe, rhubarb root, buckthorn, cascara, and castor oil. These plant-derived products have been used since ancient times for their ability to promote bowel movements and relieve constipation. Several, such as cascara, senna, and castor oil, also are available as over-the-counter drug laxatives and are regulated as drugs.

Some of these substances also are used in much smaller quantities as natural flavorings in other foods. As such, they are regulated by FDA as food additives or "generally recognized as safe" substances. FDA has not received any information suggesting that these substances pose a hazard when used in the amounts normally needed to provide flavoring.

Except when used solely as flavorings, the names of these plant substances appear in the ingredient list on the label of these products. Dieter's teas and similar products often list the substances at or near the top because they often are the main ingredients. FDA proposed in December 1995 to require manufacturers to declare dietary ingredients, including proprietary blends, in descending order of predominance by weight on product labels. In the proposed rule, the substance would have to be given by its common or usual name: for example, Tinnevelly senna followed by its Latin name, *Cassia angustifolia*.

Most consumers who use dieter's teas and similar products know that the products have laxative properties, according to health professionals familiar with the products, even though the product labeling does not specifically state the term "laxative." Instead, the labeling may promote the product as a natural bowel cleanser. Sometimes it may not reflect the laxative qualities at all.

The product labels may not directly state that the products are for weight loss, although some allude to it. For instance, some products use the terms "dieter's," "diet," "trim," or "slim" in their names. Others may carry information on weight-loss practices, mentioning consumption of the product along with the weight-loss practices. Some of the teas are labeled as "low-calorie." Unless sweetened, they provide essentially no nutrients and no calories.

> ✣ **It's A Fact!**
>
> Laxative-induced diarrhea does not significantly reduce absorption of food calories. This is because the laxatives do not work on the small intestine, where calories are absorbed, but rather on the colon, the lower end of the bowel.

According to Ara DerMarderosian, Ph.D., professor of pharmacognosy (study of medicinal products in their crude, or unprepared, form) and medicinal chemistry at the Philadelphia College of Pharmacy and Science, users favor the products because they believe that the products may cost less and taste better than over-the-counter laxatives and because they are easy to buy. In addition, he said, people with eating disorders, such as bulimia and anorexia nervosa, may like the products because they act quickly and produce loose, watery stools. Unfortunately, this practice is not only useless for losing weight but can be dangerous for people on severely restricted diets.

Writing in the January 1996 *American Druggist*, DerMarderosian and his colleague Sharon Brudnicki, a registered pharmacist also with the Philadelphia College of Pharmacy and Science, noted that some users like dieter's tea and other stimulant laxatives for their purported "body cleansing" ability.

DerMarderosian was a member of the FDA Food Advisory Committee's 1995 special task group on stimulant laxative substances in food.

Adverse Effects

Reports filed with FDA indicate that users tend to experience adverse effects when they misuse the products by, for example, steeping the tea longer than product labeling recommends or drinking more than the recommended amount. The reports indicate three types of adverse events:

- *Short-term*: stomach cramps, nausea, vomiting, and diarrhea lasting several days. These symptoms are likely to occur in first-time users who drink more than the recommended amount.

> ✔ **Quick Tip**
>
> Misuse of laxative products can result adverse effects, including nausea, vomiting, abdominal cramps, diarrhea, impaired colon function, and even death.

- *Chronic*: chronic diarrhea, pain and constipation due to laxative dependency, which causes a sluggish bowel. In one report to FDA, a person who reported using herbal products with stimulant laxatives for decades suffered severe pain and constipation from loss of colon function and required surgery to remove the colon. People who develop chronic problems usually have used these types of products for years.

- *Severe*: fainting, dehydration and electrolyte disorders (for example, low blood potassium, a condition that can cause paralysis, irregular heartbeat, and possibly death). People who develop severe problems tend to be those who are nutritionally compromised, partly as a result of drastic reductions in food intake—for example, rigorous weight-loss dieters and people with the eating disorders anorexia nervosa and bulimia. Four deaths reported to FDA involved women with a history of such medical problems. According to information presented at a 1995 meeting of FDA's Food Advisory Committee, these herbal stimulant laxatives may have been a contributing factor in their deaths.

Label Warning

At the 1995 meeting, the advisory committee's task group agreed that dietary supplements containing stimulant laxatives can have adverse effects and that a label statement would be helpful in warning consumers about the risks and reducing the incidence of these adverse effects. The group proposed this label warning:

> "NOTICE (or WARNING): Contains herbs (insert name of herbs) that can act as stimulant laxatives. Prolonged steeping time can increase the risk of adverse laxative effects, including: nausea, vomiting, abdominal cramps, and diarrhea. Chronic use of laxatives can impair colon function. Use of laxatives may be hazardous in the presence of abdominal pain, nausea, vomiting, or rectal bleeding. Laxative-induced diarrhea does not significantly reduce absorption of food calories. Acute or chronic diarrhea may result in serious injury or death."

The full advisory committee concurred with the recommendations.

California has taken steps to require a similar warning label statement on all food products containing stimulant laxatives sold in that state. Some manufacturers have begun to carry the state's drafted warning statement on their food products. FDA will monitor products sold nationally to be sure that their labels carry information similar to that required in California.

The California warning advises all users of these types of dietary supplements to:

- Read and follow package directions carefully.
- Stop using the product if diarrhea, loose stools, or stomach pain develop.
- See a doctor if frequent diarrhea develops.
- See a doctor before using the product if the user is pregnant, nursing, taking medication, or has a medical condition.

Consumer Action

Consumers should report adverse effects associated with use of laxative teas or supplements to FDA by calling FDA's MedWatch adverse event and product problem hotline at 1-800-FDA-1088. Additional information about the MedWatch program can be found at www.fda.gov/medwatch/report/consumer/consumer.htm on FDA's Website.

The report should include:

- name, address and telephone number of the person who became ill
- name and address of the doctor or hospital providing medical treatment
- description of the problem
- name of the product and store where it was bought.

Consumers also should report the problem to the manufacturer or distributor listed on the product's label and to the store where the product was bought.

🖘 Remember!

People who choose use dieter's teas should follow package directions carefully. Consumers should seek medical attention for persistent diarrhea, abdominal cramps, and other bowel problems to prevent more serious complications.

Chapter 33

Are Weight-Loss Diets Recipes For Weight Gain?

Researchers have known for decades that the effects of extreme starvation can linger. For example, Canadian prisoners starved by their German captors during World War II went through episodes of binge eating long after they had been released and restored to their normal weights.

Now scientists are finding that people who intentionally make themselves hungry by constantly going on strict diets are at the same risk of binge eating—which could help explain why many people end up weighing more after a diet than they did to begin with. Janet Polivy, PhD, a professor of psychology and psychiatry at the University of Toronto, has observed that college students who attempt to adhere to rigid dieting patterns—such as calorie counting, strict portion control, avoidance of certain foods or food groups— "bear a remarkable resemblance" in behavior to truly starved people. She calls these on-again-off-again dieters "restrained eaters."

Why Restrained Eating Backfires

Chronic dieters, or restrained eaters, train themselves to ignore their bodies' hunger signals. That leaves them susceptible to eating in response to myriad

About This Chapter: Text in this chapter is from "Are Weight-Loss Diets Recipes For Weight Gain?" in *Tufts University Diet and Nutrition Letter*, November 1996, © Tufts University. Reprinted with permission, *Tufts University Health & Nutrition Letter*, tel. 1-800-274-7581.

external signals—TV commercials for food, a bad day at work, an argument with a loved one, tiredness, boredom.

Preliminary research also indicates that dieting as a way of life may change taste perception and thereby affect how much someone eats of a particular food at a sitting. Consider

> ♣ It's A Fact!
>
> People who intentionally make themselves hungry by constantly going on strict diets are at risk of binge eating.

that, like victims of starvation and patients with anorexia nervosa, chronic dieters exhibit negative alliesthesia—a failure to reject sweet tastes just after having a sweet food. A normal eater would cross over a sweet "threshold" and not desire sugary items right after eating something sweet.

The good food/bad food mentality that is often part and parcel of restrained eaters' approach to food also influences the amount they consume. Normally, when a person eats a high-calorie snack or meal, he or she feels full and stops eating—no matter what foods the calories come from. But Dr. Polivy and others have found that when restrained eaters indulged in a calorie-dense food they perceived as bad (in this case, a milkshake), they then went overboard on other "bad" foods, including ice cream, cookies, and nuts, presumably because they felt they had "blown it" anyway. On the other hand, when the dieters ate what they considered a "good" food (a salad), they did not go on to overeat, even though the salad contained the same number of calories as the milkshake due to the addition of fat-laden dressing and other high-calorie ingredients.

✎ **Weird Words**

Alliesthesia: The perception that the same sensation is either pleasant or unpleasant depending on other factors and circumstances; sometimes the sensation is perceived as pleasant and sometimes the sensation is perceived as unpleasant.

Satiety: Eating food until one is "full"—satisfied.

Does Dieting Rule Your Life?

Has chronic dieting skewed your relationship with food, getting in the way of your body's physiologic cues of hunger and satiety—and leading to episodes of binge eating that could make you gain rather than lose or maintain your weight? To find out, answer these questions from the Restrained Eating Questionnaire, developed by Dr. Polivy and colleagues.

1. How often are you dieting?

   a. never
   b. rarely
   c. sometimes
   d. usually
   e. always

2. What is the maximum amount of weight (in pounds) you have ever lost in 1 month?

   a. 0-4
   b. 5-9
   c. 10-14
   d. 15-19
   e. 20+

3. What is your maximum weight gain (in pounds) within a week?

   a. 0-1
   b. 1-2
   c. 2-3
   d. 3-5
   e. 5+

4. In a typical week, how much does your weight (in pounds) fluctuate?

   a. 0-1
   b. 1-2
   c. 2-3
   d. 3-5
   e. 5+

5. Would a weight fluctuation of 5 pounds affect the way you live your life?

   a. not at all
   b. slightly
   c. moderately
   d. very much

6. Do you eat sensibly in front of others and splurge alone?

   a. never
   b. rarely
   c. often
   d. always

7. Do you give too much time and thought to food?

   a. never
   b. rarely
   c. often
   d. always

8. Do you have feelings of guilt after overeating?

   a. never
   b. rarely
   c. often
   d. always

9. How conscious are you of what you're eating?

   a. not at all
   b. slightly
   c. moderately
   d. very much

10. How many pounds over your desired weight were you at your maximum weight?

   a. 0-1
   b. 1-5
   c. 6-10
   d. 11-20
   e. 21+

Scoring: For every "a" answer, count 0. For a "b" answer, score 1; c, 2; d, 3; and e, 4. Add up the points. A score of 15 or more indicates that your eating patterns may be overly restrictive—like those of a restrained eater.

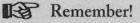 **Remember!**

Rigid dieting patterns—such as calorie counting, strict portion control, avoidance of certain foods or food groups—can lead to behaviors similar to those observed in truly starved people. This sequence of events may make some people more prone to gaining additional weight.

Chapter 34

Get Physical!

Are you getting any real exercise? If not, you may be in what fitness guru Dr. Kenneth Cooper calls "the adolescent slump." After the go-go years of childhood (remember when your day just naturally included running, jumping, wrestling, and dancing around like a nut?), studies show that many teens develop a more sit-down lifestyle. They ride in cars instead of walking. They sit and laugh at the "little kids" who still play group games out in the neighborhood. And instead of playing volleyball, football, or basketball, most teens sit on the sidelines and cheer the 10 percent to 15 percent of their peers who do compete in sports.

So, where did all those jumping, running little kids take a wrong turn? Cooper and other "kid fitness" experts say it isn't their fault—that adults focus too much on team sports and competitions and too little on keeping middle school and high school students involved in the kind of noncompetitive activities that can lead to a lifetime of fitness. In short, they say, we don't spend enough time and effort on the millions of teens who aren't "on the team." (Even basic physical education requirements are being reduced or eliminated in many high schools.)

The result? Too many active, fit children turn into less active teenagers who enter adulthood with what one expert calls a "declining fitness profile."

About This Chapter: Text in this chapter is from "What's the World's Best Exercise? It's Your Move!," by Jan Farrington in *Current Health 2*, May 1995, © 1995 Weekly Reader Corporation; reprinted with permission.

OK, so that's the bad news. And why are we telling you all this? Because you can do something about it. You can break the pattern. You can be more active, more "fit" as a teenager than you were as a child. And you can head into adult life with a "fitness profile" that's on the way up, not down. How?

Pull Up, Push Up ... and Listen Up!

Yeah, yeah, you've heard it all before. Exercise is "good for you." But do you really know why? We've got a little list....

- *Exercise Can Improve Your Athletic Performance.* A well-exercised body is more flexible, and the joints can move easily through a wider "range of motion." Combine a specific sport with a good general exercise regimen, and you'll find you have quicker reflexes, more stamina, and all the "moves" you need to play well.

- *Exercise Can Reduce the Odds of a Sports Injury.* In his *Sportswise* guide for young athletes, teen sports physician Lyle Micheli writes that "strengthening muscles enables us to resist sprains and strains ... [and] to withstand the normal trauma of contact and collision sports such as football, soccer, basketball, and hockey." If you spend most of the week as a couch potato, don't rely on practices and games alone to make you fit, says Dr. Micheli. Make time for physical activity and exercise "outside" your special sport.

- *Exercise Can Give You a Bigger, Better Heart.* Did you know that the heart of a child or adult who exercises regularly can actually get bigger? An "exercised" heart (and we mean aerobic exercise that raises the heartbeat for 20 to 30 minutes) actually may beat a little slower when

♣ It's A Fact!

84 percent of children under age 10 are involved in physical activity with some community organization—but only 32 percent of high school seniors in another survey say they play sports or exercise three or more times a week.

it's "at rest," but pumps more blood with each beat than a "lazy" heart does. At the same time, exercise can give your heart the ability to respond to high-stress situations without trouble. And exercise also increases the levels of "good" HDL cholesterol in your blood—the "Roto-Rooter" substance that helps keep your arteries clear and open.

- *Exercise Improves Mental Alertness—and May Even Help Your Grades!* Studies of Canadian and French school children over a period of years showed that students who exercised every day performed better in many of their academic subjects than their peers who had only one exercise session per week.

- *Exercising "Now" Can Mean a Healthier "Later."* Being fit in childhood and adolescence helps people fight off a host of diseases in later life, including heart disease, back pain, osteoporosis (brittle bones), diabetes, and high blood pressure. Regular moderate exercise helps the immune system ward off minor infectious diseases (colds, for instance). And in several recent studies, physically active adults (those who exercised regularly) were found to have lower death rates from several kinds of cancer.

- *Exercise Is an Effective Way to Reduce Stress, Control Depression, and Get a Better Night's Sleep.* If you're feeling down or angry, exercise can help change your mood. "I have never started a walk angry and ended up with the same feeling that I had when I began," says Casey Meyers in his book *Walking.* "You can literally walk your anger into the ground."

- *Exercise Can Boost Self-Esteem.* When you feel and look better, you feel better about yourself. You don't have to be the star of a sports team to think of yourself as a success, either. You can compete against yourself by setting exercise goals and sticking with the activities you choose: calisthenics, jogging, walking, cycling, swimming, etc.

- *Exercise Can Add Fun and Friendship to Your Life.* Fun and friendship? Those may not be the first words you think of to pair with exercise. But if you work it right, you can have fun—and get to know friends and family better. Take an exercise class with a friend. Start walking three times a week with your dog. Organize a group to enter a local

10K race—even if you aren't runners, most races will let you "fastwalk" the course together. Exercising with people you care about—minus TV sets, video games, and other distractions—can enrich the "personal" side of your life.

✎ **Weird Words**

Aerobic exercise: The word "aerobic" refers to the presence of oxygen. Aerobic exercise is exercise in which energy is produced as oxygen is metabolized. Jogging is an example.

Anaerobic exercise: The word "anaerobic" means without oxygen. Anaerobic exercises consist of short uses of energy that do not require oxygen. Weight lifting is an example.

DON'T "Go For The Burn"

Consider these four kids:

- SHE kicks, twirls, and jumps for two hours a day in an aerobic dancing class.
- HE walks 15 minutes to the supermarket instead of taking the car.
- HE and a friend often spend weekends running in marathon races—and they train long hours during the week, too.
- SHE gave up jogging last year (shin splints) and now "does the mile" in a swimming pool three times a week.

Which of these people are in tune with the latest thinking about exercise? If you guessed the hard-driving dancers and marathoners, you're out of step.

These days, the gurus of exercise are talking "moderation." Take it easier, they say. Don't go for the burn. Don't see pain as gain. Push yourself—but not too hard.

Fitness expert Dr. Kenneth Cooper and other fitness boosters want to get the word out that you DO NOT need to become a jock or a fitness fanatic to get the benefits of exercise. "Moderate exercise," says Dr. Cooper, "something as simple as walking 30 to 45 minutes a day at a brisk pace, will produce the moderate fitness level that is associated with greatly reduced risk of death."

Who gets the most from a good exercise program? Couch potatoes! "The greatest benefits achieved," says a government study, "when the least active individuals [i.e., potatoes] become moderately active." A long-term study of nearly 17,000 Harvard graduates found that health benefits—including a 20 percent the death rate!—began for those who burned as few as 500 calories a week in exercise. (Walking 15 minutes a day or playing tennis for one hour each week will burn 500 calories. The studies say that active people should stay active—but that they don't really improve health or lower the risk of death by becoming "extremely active." What's more, people who overdo exercise face a skyrocketing risk of injuries to muscles, joints, and other overused body parts.

Another 1993 report added that we should pay attention to the benefits of "real life" physical activity, too. (Your parents will LOVE this!) Dusting and vacuuming, raking leaves, washing windows, or cutting the grass is good exercise, too. We all still need a few short sessions each week (15 to 30 minutes each) of the kind of aerobic exercise that makes your heart beat fast. But in between, you can work on strength, stamina, and flexibility through exercise, sports, and other physical activities that get your body moving and working at a steady pace.

What activities? The choices are almost endless...and they're up to you! Take a look at the list of sports and activities in Table 34.1. Note things you already do at least once a week and activities you'd like to try. Be adventurous, but realistic: Some sports you may have to put off for later (surfing if you live far from the ocean, skiing if it's too expensive, etc.). Focus on things you can actually do in your own area right now.

Fitness benefits from exercise can begin for people who burn at least 500 calories per week in deliberate exercise or activity. Draw up a list of activities

✔ Quick Tip: 10 Ways To Get Physical!

1. *Take Your Feet:* Forget about asking your folks for a ride. Put your feet to the ground and start walking. Your feet will thank you, your heart will thank you, and Mother Nature will thank you for helping cut down on air pollution.

2. *Try In-line Skating:* Fun, fast, and easy to learn, in-iine skating is a great way to spend a day outside with friends. Remember to wear the gear: a helmet and knee, wrist, and elbow pads.

3. *Take the Stairs:* Forget the elevator. By simply taking the stairs every chance you can, yo u'll get a workout without even thinking.

4. *Walk the Dogs:* Whether you volunteer or get paid, dog walking is a fun, furry way to be physically active.

5. *Bike There:* Mountain bikes are it! They go wherever you take 'em. So grab your friends and hit the trail. Of course, wear a helmet.

6. *Earn Extra Cash:* That's right. Make money while helping your body. Try mowing lawns, weeding gardens, shoveling snow, and cleaning garages.

7. *Turn Up the Music:* Shake, rattle, and roll to your favorite tunes. It doesn't matter what you do as long as you move to the beat.

8. *Baby Sit:* Sounds silly, but if you've never kept up with a toddler you're in for a big surprise. They move—and they move fast! Keeping your eye on a tot can challenge even the quickest teen.

9. *Lap It Up:* Swimming, diving, even water polo are all great activities and a real splash to do with friends. So don't be a drip, learn to do a flip.

10. *Play One-On-One Basketball:* Talk about a total body workout. First person to 21 wins!!!

Source: From YourSelf, produced by the U.S. Department of Agriculture (USDA).

you could do this week to use up 500 calories. (Use the per-minute calorie count on the table that is closer to your body weight.) Then make a list of fitness activities you'd like to add on in later weeks. Visualize yourself now, and then "see" yourself after six months following this program. How do you feel? Bouncy, more energetic, better-looking? What things will you be able to do then that you can't do now? Exercise is one way you can plan to make your life better: healthier and more fun.

Fifteen to 20 minutes of exercise is as relaxing as taking a tranquilizer, say recent studies. Why? Researchers think exercise releases increased levels of natural pain killers and "mood elevators" called endorphins into the bloodstream—creating a natural feeling of well-being and calm.

Table 34.1. CALORIE BURNERS: Activities That Count

Activity	Calories Burned (per minute)	
	120 lbs.	180 lbs.
Aerobic dance	6.2	8.2
Basketball (half-court)	4.3	5.6
Bicycling (13 mph)	9.0	14.0
Canoeing (4 mph)	5.7	8.4
Dancing (rock 'n' roll)	6.0	8.0
Football (touch)	4.3	5.8
Golf (carrying clubs)	3.5	4.8
Gymnastics	4.4	6.0
Hiking	4.3	5.8
Jogging (5.5 mph)	9.2	12.5
Mowing lawn (hand mower)	4.2	5.3
Skating (ice)	5.0	6.7
Skating (roller)	5.0	6.7
Skiing (cross-country)	9.9	13.4
Soccer	7.7	10.4
Softball (fast pitch)	4.0	5.4
Swimming (50 yd. per min.)	8.8	12.6
Tennis (doubles)	4.0	16.0
Tennis (singles)	6.0	8.0
Volleyball	5.0	6.7
Walking (2 mph)	3.0	4.8
Walking (4.5 mph)	5.5	9.0
Weight training	6.7	9.0

Eeny, Meeny: More Than One ... Is Even Better!

By now you've got the idea: The world's best exercise is the one you DO! Your goal should be to get some kind of "formal" exercise three or four times a week, and to find ways to put more "informal" activity into your life. Here's how one high school girl's exercise choices shape up:

Sunday: Hiked around the lake with friends.

Monday: Exercise video (low-impact, 20 minutes plus warm-up/cool-down time).

Tuesday: Soccer practice, including laps around the field.

Wednesday: Treadmill in fitness center with Mom.

Thursday: Soccer practice.

Friday: Nothing much—but raked leaves and biked to a friend's house.

Saturday: The game. We lost, but played hard.

This girl is an athlete in training—and does more exercise than you'd need to bring yourself up to a "moderate" fitness level.

But fitness experts say this kind of varied routine is a good way to avoid boredom—and to reduce the chances of overuse injuries from working out "the same way" every time. But even if you change exercises from day to day, remember that building fitness means regular exercise sessions—three or four times a week, year-round. Why? Because your body tends to build fitness slowly, and lose it rapidly. Take one week off, for instance, and your cardio-respiratory (heart-lung) fitness will drop by 10 percent.

The best exercise "mix" often includes three somewhat different components:

- a regular set of conditioning exercises for strength and flexibility (what your grandparents might call "calisthenics").

- fun sports/activities that provide an aerobic workout: cycling, swimming, walking, tennis, rowing, dancing, and so on. (Focus on activities that make you breathe fast and keep your major muscles constantly moving and working—a sure sign that you're getting the aerobic exercise your heart and lungs need.) With a little creative thinking, you can turn some of these workouts into social occasion—for instance, turning an exercise hike and swim into a social swim and picnic by inviting a few friends along.

- more physical activity in your everyday life: tackling some of the harder aerobic housework (lawn mowing, leaf raking, window washing, etc.) ... climbing the stairs even when there's an elevator ... parking "way out" at the mall ... talking with friends while playing tennis or biking around the neighborhood, not just on the phone.

Don't know where to start? If you've been leading a fairly inactive life, start slow. Ask a friend or a favorite relative to go walking with you. Send for one of the exercise booklets listed below. Try out other activities as you go along—and don't feel guilty about dropping something that doesn't appeal

---

♣ It's A Fact!

"The percentage of teens who are overweight, which held steady at about 15 percent through the 1970s, rose to 21 percent in 1991," said a recent *Time* cover story. Studies say young Americans are eating too much fatty food and getting too little exercise. Since the 1960s, obesity has increased nearly 40 percent among 12- to 17-year-olds in the United States.

Unfortunately, some preteens and teens are endangering their health by turning to diets to control weight-while ignoring the best alternative of all: exercise. Physical activity appears to be the key to successful weight loss and maintenance," say Robert Ornstein and Dr. David Sobel in their book *Healthy Pleasures*. "Following exercise, [your body's] metabolic rate stays up for as long as 24 hours, so you may continue to burn up extra calories while relaxing after a workout." Regular exercise appears to signal your brain to reduce the amount of fat stored in your body, allowing you to lower (slowly) your overall body fat levels.

to you: There are always other options. Just be sure to choose something, and (in the words of the ad) Just Do It.

You know what exercise can do for you. You know it won't take much time out of your week to become an ex-couch potato. You know you'll feel better about yourself and your life. So ... make your move today!

☞ **Remember!**

Chances are that you will lose weight if you exercise and eat healthy. But even without the weight control benefits, exercise would still be worth it—as a way to work off stress, improve strength and stamina, and avoid health problems in your adult life. With the added benefit of proven weight control—why wouldn't you try it?

Chapter 35

How Do I Gain 10 Pounds?

Question

I see tons of information about weight loss, but I need to gain 10 pounds! At 5 feet 5 inches, I'm a scrawny 110 pounds and would feel better at 120 or so. As a woman, I'm not interested in "bulking up" either. My friends have no suggestions and tell me to get a "real" problem. But I'm tired of not filling out my clothes—they particularly sag in the rear. Please help!

Answer

Take solace in that many folks have your same problem—a desire to gain weight and not much luck finding help from friends, the Internet, or elsewhere.

It sounds like you want to put on some body fat along with a bit of muscle to fill out your pants and not feel so "scrawny." Putting on weight, whether 10 pounds or 50 pounds (as some tall, skinny men have asked about), takes three things.

1. Eating extra calories beyond what you need to maintain your weight.

2. Weight training to build up your body mass (in your case, not too much).

About This Chapter: Text in this chapter is from "How Do I Gain 10 Pounds?" by Liz Applegate, Ph.D., Nutrition and Health columnist for OnHealth at onhealth.com, © May 2000; reprinted with permission.

3. Genetic potential: Some people simply have thin body types, and their efforts to gain weight will often take longer and yield less impressive results.

With those basics in mind, let's look at how you can put on the extra padding you want. We'll start with some ways to work extra calories into your day:

- Start by checking your eating habits. You should be eating at least five to seven meals and snacks a day. Write down what you eat for three or four days to get an idea of how often you're actually stopping to take on some calories.

- Avoid skipping meals. In my experience, people who have trouble gaining weight often skip meals without realizing it. Whether you're too busy or even forget to eat, a missed meal can cost you 500 or more calories that could have gone to weight gain. Again, writing down your food intake helps keep you on track.

- Aim to eat 500 to 1,000 extra calories every day. You can usually hit this number by having a hefty snack in both the afternoon and evening: cereal and milk, peanut butter sandwich, applesauce topped with raisins and honey ...

☞ Remember!

The keys to gaining weight include:

- eating extra calories, 500 to 1,000 more than your body needs to maintain its current weight,

- weight training and exercise, and

- recognizing your genetic potential—some people simply have thin body types.

- Target energy-dense foods that pack a lot of calories into small servings. Healthy choices include avocados, nuts or nut butters, cheese, and ice cream. Warning: Cheese and ice cream are high in saturated fat, so scratch them from the list if you have risky blood cholesterol levels.

- Make sure you include quality sources of protein such as fish, soy (tofu and soy milk), lean meats, poultry, and cooked beans and grains.

As for the strength training, use light weights and do two sets of each exercise, 15 to 20 repetitions per set. Using light weights and high repetitions will keep you from building bulk. To "fill out" your rear (build up your gluteus muscle), exercises like squats and lunges work well, even with light weights or none at all.

By following these tips (and being patient for results), you'll put on a quality 10 pounds in a few months.

Part 5

Eating Disorders

Chapter 36

Eating Disorders: Perilous Compulsions

According to the American Academy of Pediatrics, 30% of American school-age children are overweight. Half of them will grow into overweight adults. Obesity is a risk factor in high blood pressure, elevated cholesterol, diabetes, some malignant tumors, and shortened lifespan.

Factors attributed to childhood obesity include poor food choices and sedentary habits. Fast food meals—often favorite choices—typically contain 40% to 50% of their calories from fat, but these foods are low in fiber, iron, and vitamins A and C. As for lack of exercise, the title of an article in a medical publication summarized the problem: "Profusion of TV produces plump couch-potato tots." By adolescence, a child has watched 15,000 hours of television, and has been exposed to 350,000 commercials, more than half of which promote highly processed food products and soft drinks.

Linked to this problem of childhood obesity are various attempts to control dietary intake. At times, well-intentioned pressures may lead to unintended and regrettable developments. Eating disorders may develop during the adolescent years.

There is an emerging preoccupation with "healthy eating" and fitness among some adolescents, especially girls, that may lead to eating disorders,

About This Chapter: Text in this chapter is from "Eating Disorders: Perilous Compulsions," by Beatrice Trum Hunter in *Consumers' Research Magazine*, September 1997, © 1997 Consumers' Research Inc.; reprinted with permission.

according to Dr. David S. Rosen, director of adolescent health at the Medical Center of the University of Michigan at Ann Arbor. According to Rosen, healthy eating for teenage girls parallels the "vilification of fat in the media and the increasing availability and aggressive marketing of low-fat and no-fat food options." Rosen observes that moderately limiting fat intake may be desirable, but when carried to an extreme, "the compulsive avoidance of fat begins to take on the characteristics of an eating disorder and probably requires the same kind of intervention."

Pressure to be thin is increasing. Over the last few decades, *Playboy* centerfold models and Miss America contestants have become leaner, with smaller busts and hips. By contrast, the average female between 17 and 24 has become heavier and heavier.

Despite the plethora of weight-reducing diets, meals-in-cans, pills, low-fat products, non-caloric sweeteners, gym equipment, exercise programs, sweat boxes, and other approaches, young people, as well as other segments of the population, are becoming more and more obese. According to the Centers for Disease Control and Prevention, Americans are more overweight now than at any time since the government began to keep complete statistics in the 1960s. At present, 14% of children aged six to 11, and 12% of those aged 12 to 17 are dangerously overweight.

Risks In Dieting

"Dieting is a chief cause of obesity in America," according to Professor Judith Rodin of Yale University. "Some middle-class parents trying to save their daughters from the stigma of fat insist on severe diets, but depriving children of food may only make them more interested in eating. At some early stage in infancy, people, as well as animals, are pretty well biologically regulated. It takes something to deregulate that system. And one of the things

♣ It's A Fact!

Crash diets, which depend on drastic calorie reduction to induce weight loss, often backfire and result in weight gain. Many crash dieters may gain back more weight than they lost on the diet.

that we know that does that is dieting. That kind of girth control begins to slow down the metabolic rate, and makes the body begin to change in order to protect itself against the reduction in calories. This causes more problems when the dieter returns to eating normally."

Weight cycling—popularly called "yo yo" dieting—attracts many young women. Studies have shown that repeated attempts to lose weight, followed by weight gains, greatly increase the risk for developing heart disease. Also, people who diet frequently may develop a preference for high-fat and sugary foods, resulting in increased weight.

Crash diets, which depend on drastic calorie reduction to induce weight loss, often backfire and result in weight gain. Severely restricted caloric intake triggers a body response that slows the rate at which calories are used for daily activities. The body adjusts itself to run on fewer calories, and it becomes more efficient in using the available calories in order to conserve its nutrient reserves. When weight loss plateaus, many dieters become frustrated and return to their previous eating habits. However, since the body has learned to function with fewer calories, it stores more calories from the regular diet in the form of fat. The initial pounds lost on a crash diet are mostly water, released by the metabolic changes that occurred as the system adapted to reduced calories. However, the pounds regained are stored as fat. The weight gain will continue until the body returns to its former rate of processing nutrients. Thus, many crash dieters may gain back more weight than they lost on the diet.

Dieting is especially common among adolescent girls and young women who typically report weight concerns and who attempt to restrict their fat or caloric intake as early as age nine or ten years. In the last few decades, the prevalence of such concerns and subsequent efforts to diet have risen dramatically. Eating disorders are now the third most common illness among adolescent females. More than one in five girls score in the abnormal range on tests of eating attitudes and behaviors, and abnormal scores are noted commonly in girls as young as fourth and fifth graders.

Although these problems are encountered mainly with females, adolescent boys and young men with severely abnormal eating habits are being identified more frequently as well.

Dieting by teenagers, from infrequent to uninterrupted, is a sign of possible eating disorders. Rosen says that eating disorders occur on a continuum, ranging from mild to serious manifestations.

Anorexia Nervosa

On the continuum of eating disorders, anorexia nervosa is in the extreme of the range. It has long been recognized as a serious health problem, thought to result from emotional or psychological stresses. The typical patient is a white middle-to-upper middle class young woman, but increasingly, cases are reported among some women of other ages, and in males, and in nonwhites.

Typically, an anorexic refuses to maintain weight that is above the lowest weight considered to be normal for her age and height. Her total body weight is at least 15% below normal. She displays an intense fear of weight gain, despite the fact that she may be severely underweight. Regarding herself in a mirror, she has a distorted image of her body and is convinced that she is fat. Frequently, she fails to menstruate. She suffers a pathological loss of appetite, accompanied by nutritional deficiency symptoms.

✎ Weird Words

Anorexia Nervosa: An eating disorder with a loss of appetite for food, characterized by a fear of gaining weight or becoming fat.

Binge Eating: An eating disorder characterized by eating large amount of food in short periods of time but without the purging associated with bulimia nervosa.

Bulimia Nervosa: An eating disorder characterized by eating large amounts of food in short time periods. One type includes self-induced vomiting or the abuse of laxatives to control weight; another type includes strict dieting, fasting, or excessive exercising.

Pica: An eating disorder characterized by persistent and compulsive cravings to eat inedible substances such as clay, dirt, cornstarch, laundry starch, baking soda, chalk, buttons, ice, paper, dried paint, cigarette butts, burnt matches, ashes, sand, soap, toothpaste, oyster shells, or even broken crockery.

Over time, vital organs such as the heart and liver may be damaged. Without intervention, there is emaciation, wasting, shrunken organs, and death.

According to governmental surveys, cases of anorexia nervosa have doubled in the past 10 years. Between 0.5% and 1.0% of women during late adolescence and early adulthood are thought to be affected. Onset may be triggered by a stressful life event, such as leaving home.

In young males, compulsive running has come to be regarded as a counterpart of anorexia nervosa in young women. Compulsive running is self-destructive and pathological behavior. It is primarily a male manifestation of what is termed an "ascetic disorder." However, there are some young women who are compulsive runners, too, but they are fewer in numbers. Like anorexics, compulsive runners tend to be high achievers from affluent families. Pathological commitment begins at a time of heightened stress. In recent years, its incidence has increased dramatically.

Anorexia is poorly understood. One theory relates this eating disorder to a malfunctioning hypothalamus, an organ that controls the release of morphine-like endorphins in response to stress. Emaciated anorexics have abnormally high brain levels of endorphins. The same brain chemistry may play a role in the emotional "high" reported by compulsive runners.

Bulimia Nervosa

Bulimia nervosa is another serious eating disorder of young people, characterized by repeated binge eating and purging. The episodes may be repeated frequently. The person—usually a young woman—consumes excessive amounts of food within a brief period of time, and then induces vomiting or uses a laxative, diuretic, or enema to get rid of the food. When not bingeing, the bulimic may adhere to a strict dieting or fasting regime, or indulge in vigorous exercise, in attempting to prevent weight gain.

Often, bulimics attempt to hide their problem. They may eat normally with other people, but binge and purge in private. Many maintain normal weight. Observant family members, college roommates, or school personnel who suspect bulimia, should look for some warning signs: a chronically inflamed

and sore throat that bleeds, decaying tooth enamel caused by frequent exposure to stomach acid that results from induced vomiting, and swollen sali-
vary glands in the neck and jaw which makes the face look puffy.

Recent studies by Christopher G. Fairburn and his associates at Oxford
University have pinpointed some of the psychological risk factors in early
childhood that can contribute to bulimia at a later stage. Frequently, at an
early age, the children had viewed themselves with extreme disdain. They
had experienced minimal contacts with their parents, or were physically or sexu-
ally abused. They encountered parental conflicts or criticisms. The parents, themselves, frequently had suffered from obesity or bouts of depression. Many of the
parents had demanded perfection. Many of the children who later developed
bulimia had wrestled with obesity early in life, or had other health problems.
Early menstruation, accompanied by body-shape changes, spurred dieting. Bouts
of depression or other mental conditions often preceded bulimia. Current dieting by other family members or their critical comments about dieting reinforced
the problem. In gathering these risk factors together, psychological components
become apparent in the origin of this eating disorder.

It is estimated that between 1% and 3% of American adolescent and young
women are bulimic. Among college-age women, the problem may affect as
many as 20%.

Little is known about the long-term prospects for recovery from bulimia,
either with or without intervention. A statistical compilation of existing data
suggests that about 50% of all women initially diagnosed with bulimia were
free of their symptoms after five to 10 years, regardless of whether or not
they received treatment. Another 20% still had the disorder. The remaining
30% continued to binge and purge, but they fell short of being classified
officially as bulimic.

According to Pamela K. Keel and James E. Mitchell of the University of
Minnesota in Minneapolis, treatment for bulimics could speed the recovery
of women who, on their own, stop bingeing and purging after five to 10
years. Nonetheless, Keel and Mitchell reported that in the first four years
after the initial bulimic diagnosis, about one-third of those who recover still
suffer relapses.

Binge Eating

Binge eating, a related eating disorder, has some features similar to bulimia, but is regarded as a distinct entity by medical doctors. Even less is known about binge eating than anorexia or bulimia. It is estimated that about 2% of the general American population is affected. Bingers may comprise about 30% of all individuals who attend weight-control programs in hospital settings. An even larger percentage of bingers may exist among some members of the population, such as obese patients who suffer from compulsive mental disorders.

Like bulimics, bingers may consume extraordinary amounts of food in a brief time, but unlike bulimics, they do not attempt to purge. After an episode of bingeing, the following morning may produce symptoms similar to those of the severe hangover of an alcoholic. The binger is rendered nonfunctional for school activities or in the workplace.

Pica

Pica, a bizarre eating disorder, has long been known. It was described in the ancient world by Hippocrates. It is known globally. Its name is derived from the Latin for magpie—a bird known for its voracious and indiscriminate appetite. Persons suffering from pica display persistent and compulsive cravings to eat inedible substances such as clay, dirt, cornstarch, laundry starch, baking soda, chalk, buttons, ice, paper, dried paint, cigarette butts, burnt matches, ashes, sand, soap, toothpaste, oyster shells, or even broken crockery.

Most frequently, pica occurs in women before or during their pregnancies or while they are nursing. However, pica has been reported in non-pregnant and non-nursing women, as well as in children, epileptics, the mentally retarded, and psychotic individuals. Sometimes, several household members share these cravings.

Eating of earth substances such as clay or dirt, known as geophagia, is a form of pica that can cause iron deficiency. It has been practiced by pregnant African-American women in the South. Some, who have migrated to the North, have arranged for regular mailings of clay dug from some favorite area. In addition, southern grocery stores have sold clay intended for human consumption. It is thought that clay eating causes iron deficiency by binding iron in the gut. Some clays have been found to decrease iron absorption by 25%. Starch eating also contributes to iron deficiency because starch lacks minerals.

Pica is a serious eating disorder that can inflict gastrointestinal problems that may require surgery, dental injury, phosphorus intoxication (from matchheads), or environmental poisoning from lead or mercury that can be contaminants in the ingested substances.

The cause(s) and prevalence of pica are unknown. Theories abound, including nutritional, sensory, physiologic, psychosocial, and cultural explanations. The most common suspected factors are emotional disturbances and malnutrition, resulting from deficiencies of dietary iron or zinc.

The nutritional theory suggests that appetite-regulating brain enzymes, altered by iron or zinc deficiency, lead to specific cravings. However, the craved items usually do not supply the lacking minerals.

A physiologic theory notes that eating clay or dirt has been used to relieve nausea, control diarrhea, increase salivation, remove toxins, and alter odor or taste perception. According to psychological theories, pica has been explained as a behavioral response to stress, a habit disorder, or a manifestation of an oral fixation.

Another explanation is that pica is a cultural feature in certain religious rites, folk medicine, and magical beliefs.

Despite the variety of suggested theories, no one of them explains all forms of pica.

Pica patients may be reluctant to disclose their cravings to an examining physician, or they may be unaware that their symptoms indicate some underlying problem. Doctors should familiarize themselves with the symptoms of this strange eating disorder. Many of the symptoms are common to other ailments, including fatigue, palpitations, lightheadedness, or shortness of breath. If pica is suspected, there may be signs of iron deficiency, including pallor, spooning of the nails (thinned nails that are concave and have raised edges), flattening of the tongue's papillae (small elevations on the tongue), and angular stomatitis (superficial erosions and fissurings at the angles of the mouth, which frequently signals riboflavin deficiency). A physician suspecting pica needs to be diligent and persistent in obtaining a medical history, and may need to enlist the help of the patient's family and friends.

Coping With Eating Disorders

Eating disorders are complex and cannot be treated solely with dietary means. Individual cases may need to address fundamental psychological, familial, societal, and cultural aspects of the disorder. The development of an eating disorder is not necessarily triggered only by a desire to be thin. Although much has been written about the role of Hollywood, professional models, and the media in presenting unrealistic body images to young people, the main cause of eating disorders is not from trying to achieve the perfect body.

According to a nutrition therapist, Amy Tuttle from the Renfrew Center in Philadelphia—a residential center for women with eating disorders—family dynamics often contribute to eating disorders. Tuttle reported that "some people with eating disorders come from enmeshed families where emotional, relational, and physical space boundaries may be blurry. This 'enmeshment' inhibits independence and the development of a separate self." Depression, anxiety, loneliness, stress, anger, troubled personal relationships may all contribute to disordered eating patterns. They need to be regarded as problems of coping, along with other problems such as compulsive gambling, or chronic alcohol or drug abuse.

Findings from recent research suggest that biochemical imbalances should be investigated as possible factors in eating disorders. Neurotransmitters such as serotonin and norepinephrine control appetite as well as mood, alertness, and sleeping patterns. Low levels of these chemicals may explain the relationship between eating disorders and depressive illness, or abnormal eating patterns.

Many American children are low in zinc, and zinc deficits are known to reduce the appetite. Some researchers believe that low zinc levels from crash dieting may play a role in anorexia nervosa, in addition to the psychological problems associated with that eating disorder.

Hormonal changes that can lead to taste aversions is another suspected factor in anorexia nervosa in some girls. Carl and Joan Gustavson from Arizona State University at Tempe conducted animal experiments over the past decade and found that male rats frequently became nauseated and developed taste aversions after they had been injected with estrogen, the female hormone. Similar reactions were experienced in estrogen-depleted female rats whose ovaries had been removed shortly after birth. The Gustavsons suggested that girls who produce low amounts of estrogen—possibly due to prenatal exposure to toxic substances—acquire a male-like estrogen sensitivity. Later, when estrogen concentrations greatly increase at puberty, these girls become anxious and develop taste aversions to foods. A vicious cycle continues. Dramatic weight loss reduces the nauseating estrogen concentration. Any weight gain from eating will lead only to increased estrogen concentration. In turn, this leads to anxiety and food aversions.

Currently, medications—especially antidepressants—commonly are prescribed for eating disorders. They should be regarded only as adjunct treatments to the more basic ones that address the multiplicity of factors. It is to be hoped that various areas of research may yield better understandings of the factors that cause eating disorders, and produce improved treatment.

🖙 Remember!

Eating disorders are complex and cannot be treated solely with dietary means. Individual cases may need to address fundamental psychological, familial, societal, and cultural aspects of the disorder.

Chapter 37

Anorexia Nervosa

What Is Anorexia Nervosa?

Anorexia nervosa is an eating problem that occurs when a person is extremely afraid of becoming overweight and therefore eats as little as possible. This condition is both a physical illness and a psychiatric illness. Hormone changes result from the low weight and low levels of body fat. In young women menstruation stops. Anorexia nervosa can be a very severe illness. Death may occur from starvation or suicide.

This illness occurs most often in young women. However, about 5% to 10% of people with anorexia nervosa are men.

How Does It Occur?

The cause of anorexia nervosa isn't clear. A contributing factor in many cultures is the emphasis on equating female beauty with thinness.

Factors that increase the risk of developing anorexia nervosa include:

- a family history of anorexia nervosa or other eating disorders
- a family or personal history of mood disorders, such as major depression and bipolar disorder (manic depression)

About This Chapter: Text is this chapter is from "Anorexia Nervosa," by Phyllis G. Cooper in *Clinical Reference Systems*, July 1, 1999, © 1999 Clinical Reference Systems; reprinted with permission.

What Are The Symptoms?

Symptoms may include:

- weight loss, usually severe
- binge eating (eating large amounts of food in a short time) and/or purging (using laxatives or making yourself throw up)
- tiredness
- depressed or anxious mood
- insomnia
- if you are a woman, a loss of your monthly periods when your weight drops below a certain level

How Is It Diagnosed?

Your doctor does a physical exam and medical history. Your doctor will investigate eating and other behavior patterns, such as:

- extreme selectiveness in choosing food that is low in calories
- binge eating
- purging, taking laxatives
- ritualistic eating
- overexercising
- denial of hunger and denial of any problem at all

♣ It's A Fact!

While anorexia most commonly begins in the teens, it can start at any age and has been reported from age 5 to 60. Incidence among 8 to 11-year-olds is said to be increasing.

Anorexia may be a single, limited episode with large weight loss within a few months followed by recovery. Or it may develop gradually and persist for years. The illness may go back and forth between getting better and getting worse. Or it may steadily get worse.

Anorectics may exercise excessively. Their preoccupation with food usually prompts habits such as moving food about on the plate and cutting it into tiny pieces to prolong eating, and not eating with the family.

Obsessed with weight loss and fear of becoming fat, anorectics see normal folds of flesh as "fat" that must be eliminated. When the normal fat padding is lost, sitting or lying down brings discomfort not rest, making sleep difficult. As the disorder continues, victims may become isolated and withdraw from friends and family.

Source: U.S. Food and Drug Administration, Publication No. (FDA) 96-1194, September 1997.

How Is It Treated?

This can be a very difficult condition to treat. Individual psychotherapy and family therapy are usually necessary. Medication (especially medication effective in mood disorders) may be prescribed to help reduce the fear of becoming fat, reduce depression and anxiety, and aid in weight gain. You may need to be hospitalized if your condition is severe and life-threatening.

How Long Will The Problem Last?

If you have anorexia, you may have symptoms for many years and will probably need ongoing treatment. Any stressful situation can cause a relapse. After you have reached a normal weight, you may need to continue psychotherapy or medication for months or years. In addition, you may be weighed regularly to make sure you continue eating properly.

How Can I Take Care Of Myself?

In addition to following your doctor's treatment plan and developing a support network, you can:

- Eat a nutritious, well-balanced diet.

- Moderate your exercise program.

- Get plenty of rest and sleep.

- Maintain a realistic weight for your height and body frame.

- Take mineral and vitamin supplements.

- See your doctor regularly to have your weight checked.

- Keep an optimistic outlook.

- With your therapist, work out areas of conflict in your life.

- Balance your work with recreation and social activities.

- Learn to communicate your feelings.

♣ It's A Fact!

According to statistics compiled by the American Anorexia/Bulimia Association, approximately 1,000 women die of anorexia each year.

What Can Be Done To Help Prevent Anorexia Nervosa And Maintain Good Physical Health?

Acceptance of yourself and your body can help prevent this problem. In addition you can:

- Keep appointments with your doctor or therapist.

- Avoid skipping meals.

- Avoid using laxatives.

- Avoid drinking alcohol.

- Avoid smoking cigarettes.

> ✔ **Quick Tip**
>
> Early treatment for anorexia is vital. As the disorder becomes more entrenched, its damage becomes less reversible.

☞ **Remember!**

If you think a friend of family member has anorexia, point out in a caring, nonjudgmental way the behavior you have observed and encourage the person to get medical help. If you think you have anorexia, remember that you are not alone and that this is a health problem that requires professional help. As a first step, talk to your parents, family doctor, religious counselor, or school counselor or nurse.

Source: U.S. Food and Drug Administration, Publication No. (FDA) 96-1194, September 1997.

Chapter 38

Bulimia Nervosa

What Is Bulimia?

Bulimia nervosa is an eating disorder. It is characterized by binge eating (eating large amounts of food in a short time) followed by self-induced vomiting and/or use of laxatives.

Although most bulimics have a normal weight, they feel a lack of control over their eating behavior. After bingeing, they induce vomiting or use laxatives or diuretics because they are fearful of becoming overweight. They often feel that their lives are controlled by conflicts about eating. Although the disorder can affect men, most people with bulimia nervosa are female adolescents or young women.

How Does It Occur?

The exact cause of bulimia nervosa is not known. Some researchers believe that eating disorders may be related to malfunctioning of the part(s) of the brain regulating mood and appetite.

Factors that increase the risk of developing bulimia nervosa include:

• a family history of bulimia nervosa or eating disorders

About This Chapter: Text in this chapter is from "Bulimia Nervosa," by Phyllis G. Cooper in *Clinical Reference Systems*, July 1, 1999, © 1999 Clinical Reference Systems Ltd.; reprinted with permission.

• a family or personal history of mood disorders, such as major depression or bipolar disorder (manic depression)

What Are The Symptoms?

Symptoms of bulimia include:

• repeated episodes of binge eating

• strict dieting or fasting

• repeated weight loss and gain of more than 10 pounds

• dehydration

• weakness

• depression and guilt after binge eating

• damaged teeth from gastric acid contained in vomit

• swollen cheeks from repeated vomiting

• preoccupation with being thin

• depressed or anxious mood

How Is It Diagnosed?

The doctor takes a medical history and does a physical exam. The doctor will ask about eating patterns, looking for such behavior as:

❖ It's A Fact!

Many people with bulimia maintain a nearly normal weight. Though they appear healthy and successful, in reality, they have low self-esteem and are often depressed. They may exhibit other compulsive behaviors. For example, one physician reports that a third of his bulimia patients regularly engage in shoplifting and that a quarter of the patients have suffered from alcohol abuse or addiction at some point in their lives.

Source: U.S. Food and Drug Administration, Publication No. (FDA) 96-1194, September 1997.

• repeated episodes of binge eating followed by self-induced vomiting or use of laxatives

• alternate bingeing and fasting

• secret eating and bingeing

• exercising excessively to prevent weight gain

How Is It Treated?

People with this problem must recognize that they are suffering from a dangerous disorder. Treatment involves regulation of new eating habits. The doctor may recommend psychotherapy and family counseling and may prescribe medication used for mood disorders, such as antidepressants or mood stabilizers.

♣ It's A Fact!

Studies indicate that by their first year of college, 4.5 to 18 percent of women and 0.4 percent of men have a history of bulimia.

♣ It's A Fact!

Extreme purging rapidly upsets the body's balance of sodium, potassium, and other chemicals. This can cause fatigue, seizures, irregular heartbeat, and thinner bones. Repeated vomiting can damage the stomach and esophagus (the tube that carries food to the stomach), make the gums recede, and erode tooth enamel. (Some patients need all their teeth pulled prematurely). Other effects include various skin rashes, broken blood vessels in the face, and irregular menstrual cycles.

Source: U.S. Food and Drug Administration, Publication No. (FDA) 96-1194, September 1997.

How Long Will The Effects Last?

The risk of relapse exists for years after treatment ends. Without treatment, a person with bulimia may become depressed and suicidal.

How Can I Take Care Of Myself?

- Eat well-balanced, nutritious meals.

- Schedule meals regularly, but not too rigidly. Avoid irregular eating habits and avoid fasting.

- Take vitamin and mineral supplements.

- Avoid using laxatives and diuretics.

- Seek professional help if you need to lose weight so you can lose weight slowly and to a reasonable level.

- Exercise regularly and in moderation.

What Can Be Done To Help Prevent Bulimia?

Many bulimics do not feel good about themselves. You can raise your self-esteem and thus prevent or minimize bulimia if you:

- Try to resolve areas of conflict in your life.

- Try to achieve a balance of work, social activities, recreation, rest, and exercise in your life.

- Create a support group of good friends.

- Keep a positive outlook on life.

- Stop judging yourself and others.

☞ Remember!

Most people find it difficult to stop their bulimic behavior without professional help. Early treatment is vital. If untreated, the disorder may become chronic and lead to severe health problems, even death.

If you think a friend of family member has bulimia, point out in a caring, nonjudgmental way the behavior you have observed and encourage the person to get medical help. If you think you have bulimia, remember that you are not alone and that this is a health problem that requires professional help. As a first step, talk to your parents, family doctor, religious counselor, or school counselor or nurse.

Source: U.S. Food and Drug Administration, Publication No. (FDA) 96-1194, September 1997.

Chapter 39

Binge Eating Disorder

Carol C., a 35-year-old purchasing manager, says that in a single 90-minute sitting she could eat a large mushroom pizza, 3 cheese sandwiches, a pint of chocolate ice cream, and 5 large pieces of cake smothered with frosting. Such binges became habitual, occurring as often as every other day and causing the 5'7" woman's weight to climb to 203 pounds. "I hated myself," she says. "I felt so depressed for becoming obese and not being able to control my eating. My depression would lead me to binge more, which made me feel even more guilty. It became a downward spiral."

John S., a 66-year-old retired teacher who has been bingeing since childhood, describes feeling out of control once he embarks on an eating spree. "It's like a rolling snowball," he says.

Echoing a common theme among people who binge, John says his episodes are often triggered by emotional upsets. Once, after a disturbing phone call, he ate half a box of crackers with 5 ounces of cheddar cheese, 5 tablespoons of peanut butter on 4 Wasa Toast, 2 candy bars, and 3 raspberry-filled sandwich cookies.

Almost everyone splurges now and then, often in response to stress or boredom. But what distinguishes Carol's and John's binges from garden-variety

About This Chapter: Text in this chapter is from "Binge Eating Disorder Comes Out Of The Closet: Experts Say Leading Obesity Factor Has Long Been Overlooked, in *Tufts University Diet and Nutrition Letter*, January 1997, © 1997 Tufts University. Reprinted with permission, *Tufts University Health & Nutrition Letter*, tel. 1-800-274-7581.

✤ It's A Fact!

Survey after survey has shown that Americans embrace a good-food/bad-food mentality, which holds that french fries, ice cream, and candy are "bad," as is the person who eats them. Psychologists at Arizona University underscored the point when they asked students to rate 2 hypothetical people with the exact same height, weight, and exercise habits. One of these fictitious people ate fatty foods like donuts, while the other ate so-called healthy foods like fruits and vegetables. The result the "healthy" eater was rated as more attractive, likable, hard-working, practical, and methodical than the "bad" eater.

This kind of thinking about food may be key to the core belief system of people with binge eating disorder. In fact, BED sufferers often perceive food with black-or-white thinking. After eating a piece of cake, for example, a person with BED might think "I was bad. I have no will power." This triggers feelings of distress, inadequacy, and the now-that-I've-blown-it-I-might-as-well-eat-more syndrome.

Among people with BED, all-or-nothing thinking tends to go beyond the food pantry. There also is no middle ground in relationships or in life's everyday ups and downs. For instance, instead of dealing with problems at work and recognizing that a little day-to-day conflict with others is normal, bingers often view everyday problems as catastrophes. Overwhelmed with anxiety, their feelings of inadequacy intensify.

For example, after arguing with a co-worker, a BED sufferer might tell himself, "The argument was all my fault. I'll never get anywhere in my career." This self-attack provokes such severe feelings of discomfort and anxiety that he might begin bingeing.

overeating is that the splurges become compulsive, habitual attempts to cope with life's everyday anxieties. What's more, the binges become a source of extreme guilt and shame. Many sufferers resort to such measures as bingeing alone in the car to hide their "secret" from even close friends and family.

Well-informed health experts now recognize that frequent bingeing, dubbed binge eating disorder (BED), requires psychological intervention. But BED still is not officially singled out as an eating disorder on a par with anorexia nervosa and bulimia in the latest edition of the *Diagnostic and Statistical Manual*, the "bible" of the American Psychiatric Association.

The failure to recognize that BED is a psychiatric disorder rather than a dietary one is a major obstacle standing in the way of its diagnosis and treatment, perpetuating a widespread public health problem. As many as 50 percent of obese people who seek treatment for weight loss may suffer from binge eating. About a third of these bingers are men.

"My patients tell me, 'I feel as out of control as a bulimic, but I don't purge. I wish I did purge, because then I could get treatment,'" says Seda Ebrahimi, PhD, director of the eating disorders treatment program at McLean Hospital in Belmont, Massachusetts. The lack of purging—vomiting, abusing laxatives, or overexercising after eating—is what often leads patients and physicians to overlook BED and minimize the severity of the problem, treating it simply as overeating.

Coming To Terms With BED

The definition of binge eating disorder includes the following:

- Binges occur, on average, at least twice a week for 6 months. The amount of food that constitutes a binge varies from person to person, but it generally adds up to much more than most people would eat within an hour or two. Many BED sufferers, for instance, consume as much as 10,000 calories in one sitting. Equally significant, the binger feels out of control, that he or she cannot stop eating or curb the amount eaten. During the binge, the person "mentally and emotionally checks out," according to Dr. Ebrahimi.

- A bingeing episode is associated with at least 3 of the following characteristics:

  - eating much more rapidly than normal

  - eating until feeling uncomfortably full

  - eating large amounts when not physically hungry

  - eating alone as a result of embarrassment about the amount eaten

  - feeling disgusted, depressed, or guilty afterward

> ✔ **Quick Tip**
>
> Therapy can help people recognize stressful events that may "trigger" a binge and come up with alternatives to eating, like taking a walk, calling a friend, or writing down feelings.

Extreme distress in the aftermath of a binge is one of the key hallmarks that separates BED from ordinary overeating. In fact, many BED patients wake up the day after a binge with what they call a food hangover. "It's very much like one feels after drinking too much alcohol," says Dr. Ebrahimi. "Patients feel groggy, and they cannot think clearly. They also feel physically uncomfortable."

"After a typical binge, I would feel horrible," says Carol C. "My stomach would ache and I would feel swollen. I would feel so emotionally and physically devastated that it became hard for me to go to work."

The binge is not followed by behavior to make up for the extra calories consumed, such as self induced vomiting, taking laxatives, fasting, or exercising excessively. Because the bingeing is unaccompanied by, say, throwing up or laxative abuse, people with BED tend to be obese. (On the other hand, people with bulimia are typically slender to normal weight.) The excess weight compounds feelings of low self-esteem, depression, and isolation often experienced by bingers.

Getting To The Root Of The Problem

While scientists aren't sure what causes BED, studies show that bingers tend to have a striking pattern of depression. Because the depression and bingeing are closely linked, says Dr. Ebrahimi, it's difficult to tell whether the depression causes the bingeing, or vice versa.

Anxiety and panic disorders occur relatively often in bingers. Some research also indicates that drug, alcohol, and sexual abuse are particularly prevalent among people with BED, although those associations remain tenuous.

Because depression is a major issue for many people with BED, antidepressant medications like Prozac are often prescribed shortly after diagnosis. Once the depression begins to lift, a BED sufferer can start working to figure out why the binges take place and can then try to devise strategies to control the disorder.

For John S., food is a crutch. "I use it to work through any emotional distress, whether from sexual frustration, anger, depression, rejection, fatigue, or even boredom," he says. Therapy helps people like John recognize a binge "trigger," like an argument with a co-worker, and come up with an alternative to eating, like taking a walk, calling a friend, or writing down his feelings.

Mental health experts do not encourage weight loss until the bingeing problem is tackled and under control. It is at that point that patients can begin to focus on developing healthful, moderate eating habits and losing excess pounds.

After getting her binges under control, Carol C., for example, lost 30 pounds in about 5 months. What's more, she developed healthful lifestyle habits. One is walking on a treadmill for 45 minutes several times a week, which she says helps her "blow off steam." That in turn allows her to resist the urge to binge. Whereas Carol used to be unable to eat just one piece of cake without then scarfing down the entire cake, she now can have one serving and put down her fork. Such successful results usually require professional assistance.

🖘 Remember!

Almost everyone splurges now and then, but what distinguishes binge eating disorder (BED) from garden-variety overeating is that the splurges become compulsive, habitual attempts to cope with life's everyday anxieties and the binges become a source of guilt and shame. Well-informed health experts now recognize that (BED) requires psychological intervention.

Part 6

If You Need More Information

Chapter 40

Directory Of Resources

The following organizations can provide additional information on topics related to diet, nutrition, food supplements, food allergies, and eating disorders. For your convenience in locating contact information for specific organizations, they are listed alphabetically.

American Academy of Allergy, Asthma and Immunology
611 East Wells Street
Milwaukee, WI 53202
Phone: (414) 272-6071
Toll Free: 1-800-822-2762
Fax: (414) 272-6070
E-Mail: nab@aaaai.org
Internet: http://www.aaaai.org

American Academy of Dermatology
930 N. Meacham Rd.
Schaumburg, IL 60173
Phone: (847) 330-0230
Toll Free: 1-888-462-DERM
Internet: http://www.aad.org

American Anorexia/Bulimia Association, Inc.
1165 West 46th Street, Suite 1108
New York, NY 10036
Phone: (212) 575-6200
Internet: http://www.aabainc.org

American College of Allergy, Asthma and Immunology
85 W. Algonquin Road, Suite 550
Arlington Heights, IL 60005
Toll Free: 1-800-842-7777
E-Mail: mail@acaai.org
Internet: http://allergy.mcg.edu

American College of Sports Medicine
401 W. Michigan St.
Indianapolis, IN 46202-3233
Phone: (317) 637-9200
Fax: (317) 634-7617
E-Mail: atrobec@acsm.org
Internet: http://www.acsm.org

American Dietetic Association
216 W. Jackson Blvd.
Chicago, IL 60606-6995
Phone: (312) 899-0040 x5000
Toll Free: 1-800-877-1655 Consumer Nutrition Hotline
E-Mail: cdr@eatright.org
Internet: http://www.eatright.org

American Heart Association National Center
7272 Greenville Avenue
Dallas, TX 75231-4596
Toll Free: 1-800-AHA-USA1
Internet: http://
www.americanheart.org

American Red Cross
431 18th Street, NW
Washington, DC 20006
Phone: (202) 639-3520
E-Mail: info@usa.redcross.org
Internet: http://www.redcross.org

Asthma and Allergy Foundation of America
1233 20th Street, N.W., Suite 402
Washington, DC 20036
Toll Free: 1-800-7-ASTHMA
Fax: (202) 466-8940
E-Mail: info@aafa.org
Internet: http://www.aafa.org

The Blonz Guide to Nutrition
Internet: http://blonz.com

Center for Science in the Public Interest
1875 Connecticut Ave., N.W., Suite 300
Washington, DC 20009-5728
Phone: (202) 332-9110
Fax: (202) 265-4954
E-Mail: cspi@cspinet.org
Internet: http://www.cspinet.org

Centers for Disease Control and Prevention
1600 Clifton Road
Atlanta, GA 30333
Toll Free: 1-800-311-3435
Internet: http://www.cdc.gov

Children's Nutrition Research Center
Public Affairs Office
1100 Bates St.
Houston, TX 77030
Phone: (713) 798-6782
Fax: (713) 798-7098
E-Mail: cnrc@bcm.tmc.edu
Internet: http://www.bcm.tmc.edu/cnrc

Consumer Information Center
Dept. WWWW
Pueblo, CO 81009
Phone: (202) 501-1794
Toll Free: 1-888-878-3256
Fax: (719) 948-9724
E-Mail: catalog.pueblo@gsa.gov
Internet: http://www.pueblo.gsa.gov

Dairy Council of California
1101 National Drive, Suite B
Sacramento, CA 95834
Toll Free: 1-888-868-3083 (Outside California)
Toll Free: 1-888-868-3133 (In California)
E-Mail: info@dairycouncilofca.org
Internet: http://www.dairycouncilofca.org

Eczema Association
1220 S.W. Morrison, Suite 433
Portland, OR 97205
Phone: (503) 228-4430
Toll Free: 1-800-818-7546
Fax: (503) 224-3363
E-Mail: nease@teleport.com
Internet: http://www.eczema-assn.org

Food Allergy Network
10400 Eaton Place, Suite 107
Fairfax, VA 22030-2008
Toll Free: 1-800-929-4040
Fax: (703) 691-2713
E-Mail: fan@worldweb.net
Internet: http://www.foodallergy.org

Food Marketing Institute
655 15th Street, NW
Washington, DC 20005
Phone: (202) 452-8444
Fax: (202) 429-4519
E-Mail: fmi@fmi.org
Internet: http://www.fmi.org

Healthfinder®—Gateway to Reliable Consumer Health Information
National Health Information Center
U.S. Department of Health and Human Services
P.O. Box 1133
Washington, DC 20013-1133
Phone: (301) 565-4167
Toll Free: 1-800-336-4797
Fax: (301) 984-4256
E-Mail: nhicinfo@health.org
Internet: http://www.healthfinder.gov

International Food Information Council Foundation
P.O. Box 65708
Washington, DC 20035
1100 Connecticut Ave., NW
Suite 430
Washington, DC 20036
E-mail: foodinfo@ific.health.org
Internet: http://ificinfo.health.org

Iowa State University, University Extension
Food Science and Human
Nutrition Extension
1127 Human Nutritional
Sciences Bldg.
Iowa State University
Ames, IA 50011-1120
Internet: http://
www.exnet.iastate.edu/Pages/
families/fshn

The Kellogg's Nutrition University
P.O. Box CAMB
Battle Creek, MI 49016-1986
Toll Free: (800) 962-1413
Internet: http://
www.kelloggsnu.com

National Arthritis, Musculo-skeletal and Skin Diseases Information Clearinghouse
One AMS Circle
Bethesda, MD 20892-3675
Phone: (301) 495-4484
Internet: http://www.nih.gov/niams

National Association of Anorexia Nervosa and Associated Disorders
P.O. Box 7
Higland Park, IL 60035
Phone: (847) 831-3438
Fax: (847) 433-4632
E-Mail: info@anad.org
Internet: http://www.anad.org

National Cholesterol Education Program
NHLBI/OPEC
31 Center Drive, MSC2480
Room 4A-16
Bethesda, MD 20892-2480
Phone: (301) 496-1051
Fax: (301) 402-1051
E-Mail:
NHLBIinfo@rover.nhlbi.nih.gov
Internet: http://www.nhlbi.nih.gov

National Council For Reliable Health Information
P.O. Box 1276
Loma Linda, CA 92354
Phone: (909) 824-4690
Internet: http://www.ncrhi.org

National Digestive Diseases Information Clearinghouse
2 Information Way
Bethesda, MD 20892-3570
Phone: (301) 654-3810
Fax: (301) 907-8906
E-Mail: nddic@info.niddk.nih.gov
Internet: http://
www.niddk.nih.gov/health/digest/
nddic.htm

The National Eating Disorders Organization
445 E. Greenville Road
Washington, Ohio 43085
Phone: (918) 481-4044

National Heart, Lung, and Blood Institute (NHLBI) Information Center
P.O. Box 30105
Bethesda, MD 20824-0105
Phone: (301) 592-8573
Fax: (301) 592-8563
E-Mail: nhlbiinfo@rover.nhlbi.nih.gov
Internet: http://www.nhlbi.nih.gov

National Institute of Diabetes and Digestive and Kidney Diseases
Office of Communications and
Public Liaison
31 Center Drive, MSC 2560
Bethesda, MD 20892-2560
Internet: http://www.niddk.nih.gov

National Osteoporosis Foundation
1232 22nd Street N.W.
Washington, DC 20037-1292
Phone: (202) 233-2226
Internet: http://www.nof.org

Osteoporosis and Related Bone Diseases—National Resource Center
1232 22nd Street, N.W.
Washington, DC 20037-1292
Phone: (202) 223-0344
Toll Free: 1-800-624-BONE
TTY: (202) 466-4315
Fax: (202) 293-2356
TDD: (202) 466-4315
E-Mail: arbdnrc@nof.org
Internet: http://www.osteo.org

President's Council on Physical Fitness and Sports
200 Independence Ave. S.W.
Humphrey Building, Room 738 H
Washington, DC 20001
Phone: (202) 690-9000
Fax: (202) 690-5211

Tufts University Health and Nutrition Letter
P.O. Box 420235
Palm Coast, FL 32142-0235
Phone: 1-800-274-7581
Internet: http://
www.healthletter.tufts.edu

U.S. Department of Agriculture (USDA)

Center for Nutrition Policy and Promotion
Suite 200 North Lobby
1120 20th Street, NW
Washington, DC 20036-3406
Phone: (202) 418-2312
Fax: (202) 208-2322
Internet: http://www.usda.gov/cnpp

Food and Nutrition Information Center
National Agricultural Library
Agricultural Research Service, USDA
10301 Baltimore Ave., Room 304
Beltsville, MD 20705-2351
Phone: (301) 436-7725
Internet: http://www.nal.usda.gov/fnic

Food and Nutrition Service
3101 Park Center Dr., Room 819
Alexandria, VA 22302
Phone: (703) 305-2286
E-Mail: webmaster@fns.usda.gov
Internet: http://www.fns.usda.gov/
fns

Food Safety and Inspection Service
(FSIS)
Food Safety Education and Com-
munications Staff, Room 1175-
South Bldg.
1400 Independence Ave. SW,
Washington DC 20250.
Phone: (202) 720-7943
Toll Free: 1-800-535-4555 Meat &
Poultry Hotline
E-Mail: fsis.webmaster@usda.gov
Internet: http://www.fsis.usda.gov

Nutrient Data Laboratory
USDA Agricultural Research
Service
Beltsville Human Nutrition Re-
search Center
10300 Baltimore Avenue
Building 005, Room 107, BARC-
West
Beltsville, MD 20705-2350
Phone: (301) 504-0630
Fax: (301) 504-0632
E-Mail: ndlinfo@rbhnrc.usda.gov
Internet: http://www.nal.usda.gov/
fnic/foodcomp

Team Nutrition
Internet: http://fns1.usda.gov/tn

U.S. Federal Trade Commission
(FTC)
Public Reference Branch
6th and Pennsylvania Avenue, NW
Room 130
Washington, DC 20580
Phone: (202) 326-2222
TDD: (202) 326-2502
Internet: http://www.ftc.gov

U.S. Food and Drug
Administration (FDA)
200 C Street, S.W.
Washington, DC 20204
Toll Free: 1-888-463-6332
Internet: http://www.fda.gov

Office of Consumer Affairs
HFE-88
Rockville, MD 20857
Toll Free: 1-800-FDA-4010 Food
Information Line
Phone: (202) 205-4314 in the
Washington, D.C., area

Center for Biologics Evaluation and
Research
1401 Rockville Pike, Suite 200N
Rockville, MD 20852-1448
Toll Free: 1-800-835-4709
Internet: http://www.fda.gov/cber

*Center for Food Safety and Applied
Nutrition*
200 C Street S.W.
Washington, DC 20204
Toll Free: 1-800-332-4010 FDA
Food Information and Seafood
Hotline
Internet: http://vm.cfsan.fda.gov

**University of Maryland
Cooperative Extension Service**
Publications Office, Symons Hall
University of Maryland at College
Park
College Park, MD 20742
Internet: http://
www.agnr.umd.edu/CES/Pubs/
newsletters.html#nut

**University of Minnesota, Depart-
ment of Food Science and Nutrition**
Nutritionist's Tool Box
1334 Eckles Ave.
Saint Paul, MN 55108
Phone: (612) 624-1290
Internet: http://www.fsci.umn.edu/
tools.htm

**Weight-Control Information
Network (WIN)**
1 WIN Way
Bethesda, MD 20892-3665
Phone: (202) 828-1025
Toll Free number: 1-800-946-8098
Fax: (202) 828-1028
E-mail: WIN@info.niddk.nih.gov
Internet: http://
www.niddk.nih.gov/health/nutrit/
win.htm

Chapter 41

Additional Reading

The resources listed contain accurate nutrition information and are available nationwide. Opinions expressed in the publications do not necessarily reflect the views of the U.S. Department of Agriculture [or the views of Omnigraphics, Inc.]. Your local library or bookstore can help you locate these books and journals. Other items can be obtained from the source listed.

General Nutrition Books (in alphabetical order)

The American Dietetic Association's Complete Food & Nutrition Guide, by Roberta Larson Duyff, Minneapolis, MN: Chronimed Publishing, 1996. 619 pp.

Beyond Food Labels: Eating Healthy with the % Daily Values, by Roberta Schwartz Wennik, New York: Berkley Pub. Group, 1996. 398 pp.

Complete Book of Vitamins & Minerals, by the Editors of *Consumer Guide*; contributing writers: Arline McDonald, Annette Natow, Jo-Ann Heslin, and Susan Male Smith, Lincolnwood, IL: Publications International, 1996. 560 pp.

Cut the Fat!: More than 500 Easy and Enjoyable Ways to Reduce the Fat from Every Meal, by The American Dietetic Association, New York: HarperPerennial, 1996. 211 pp.

About This Chapter: The documents cited in this chapter were excerpted from "Sensible Nutrition Resource List for Consumers," U.S. Department of Agriculture (USDA) August 1998 at http://www.nal.usda.gov/fnic/.

Eat for the Health of It, by Martha A. Erickson, Lancaster, PA: Starburst Publishers, 1997. 317 pp.

Encyclopedia of Vitamins, Minerals and Supplements, by Tova Navarra and Myron A. Lipkowitz, New York: Facts on File, 1996. 281 pp.

Nutrition for Dummies, by Carol Ann Rinzler, Chicago, IL: IDG Books Worldwide, 1997. 410 pp.

Nutrition in Women's Health, by Debra A. Krummel and Penny M. Kris-Etherton (editors), Gaithersburg, MD: Aspen Publishers, 1996. 582 pp.

Personal Nutrition, by Marie A. Boyle and Gail Zyla, Minneapolis: West Pub. Co., 1996.

Safe Food for You and Your Family, by Mildred M. Cody; The American Dietetic Association, Minneapolis, MN: Chronimed Publishing, 1996. 151 pp.

Shopping for Health: A Nutritionist's Aisle-by-Aisle Guide to Smart, Low-fat Choices at the Supermarket, by Suzanne Havala, New York: HarperPerennial, 1996. 309 pp.

The Stanford Life Plan for a Healthy Heart, by Helen Cassidy Page, John Speer Schroeder, and Tara C. Dickson, San Francisco, CA: Chronicle Books, 1996. 595 pp.

The Tufts University Guide to Total Nutrition, 2nd edition, by Stanley N. Gershoff, Catherine Whitney, and the Editorial Advisory Board of the *Tufts University Health & Nutrition Letter*, New York: HarperPerennial, 1996. 342 pp.

The Vegetarian Handbook. Eating Right for Total Health, by Gary Null, New York, NY: St. Martin's Griffin, 1996. 303 pp.

Vitamins, Minerals and Food Supplements, by Marsha Hudnall, Minneapolis, MN: Chronimed Publishing, 1996. 167 pp.

Food Composition Books (in alphabetical order)

Bowes & Church's Food Values of Portions Commonly Used, 17th edition, revised, by Jean A.T. Pennington, Philadelphia, PA: J.B. Lippincott, 1998. 481 pp.

The Complete Book of Food Counts, by Corinne T. Netzer, New York, NY: Dell Publishing, 1997. 770 pp.

The Complete Food Count Guide, by the Editors of *Consumer Guide,* with the Nutrient Analysis Center, Chicago Center for Clinical Research, Lincolnwood, IL: Publications, Ltd., 1996. 704 pp.

The Complete and Up-To-Date Fat Book. A Guide to the Fat Calories, and Fat Percentages in Your Food, by Karen J. Bellerson, New York, NY: Avery Publishing Group, 1997. 870 pp.

Fast Food Facts. The Original Guide for Fitting Fast Food into a Healthy Lifestyle, by Marion J. Franz, MS, RD, LD, CDE, Minneapolis, MN: IDC Publishing, 1998. 243 pp.

The Fat Counter. The Revised and Updated 4th edition, by Annette B. Natow and Jo-Ann Heslin, New York, NY: Pocket Books, 1998. 661 pp.

Magazines/Newsletters (in alphabetical order)

Cooking Light. Southern Living, Inc., P.O. Box C-549, Birmingham, AL 35282-9990. (800) 336-0125.

Eating Well: The Magazine of Food and Health. P.O. Box 1001, Charlotte, VT 06446. (800) 344-3350.

Environmental Nutrition. P.O. Box 420235, Palm Coast, FL 32142-0235. (800) 829-5384.

Mayo Clinic Health Letter. Subscription Services, P.O. Box 53889, Boulder, CO 80322-3889. (800) 333-9037.

Nutrition Action Healthletter. Center for Science in the Public Interest (CSPI), 1875 Connecticut Ave., NW, Suite 300, Washington, DC 20009-5728. (202) 332-9110.

Tufts University Health & Nutrition Letter. P.O. Box 420235, Palm Coast FL 32142-0235. (800) 274-7581.

University of California at Berkeley Wellness Letter. Health Letter Associates, P.O. Box 420-235, Palm Coast, FL 32142-0235. (800) 829-9080.

Booklets/Pamphlets (in alphabetical order)

Available from the **American Dietetic Association**, 216 West Jackson Blvd., Suite 800, Chicago, IL 60606-6995. (312) 899-0040 or (800) 877-1655 Toll Free:

- "Food Strategies for Men" (1997)

- "Good Nutrition Reading List" (1996)

- "The New Cholesterol Countdown" (1997)

- "Staying Healthy—A Guide for Elder Americans" (1997)

Available from the **American Heart Association**, National Center, 7272 Greenville Ave., Dallas, TX 75231-4596. (800) AHA-USA1:

- "Easy Food Tips for Heart Healthy Eating" (1996)

- "AHA Diet, An Eating Plan for Healthy Americans" (1996)

- "Nutritious Nibbles: A Guide to Healthy Snacking" (1996)

Available from the **American Institute for Cancer Research**, Attn: Publications Department, 1759 R Street, NW, Washington, DC 20009. Designate Agency #0808. (202) 843-8114, http://www.aicr.org/form1.htm:

- "AICR Diet and Health Guidelines for Cancer Prevention" (1998)

- "Cooking Solo" (1996)

- "Healthy Flavors of the World: India" (1997)

- "Healthy Flavors of the World: Mediterranean" (1997)

- "No Time to Cook" (1998)

Available from the **Consumer Information Center**, Pueblo, CO 81009. (888) 878-3256, Fax: (719) 948-9724, Internet: http://www.pueblo.gsa.gov:

- "Critical Steps Towards Safer Seafood" (1997)
- "Fight BAC! Four Simple Steps to Food Safety" (1998)
- "Fruits & Vegetables: Eating Your Way to 5 a Day" (1997)
- "Growing Older, Eating Better" (1997)
- "How to Help Avoid Foodborne Illness in the Home" (1997)
- "A Pinch of Controversy Shakes Up Dietary Salt" (1997)

Available from **Iowa State University, Cooperative Extension Services**, Publication Distribution Printing & Pub. Bldg., Iowa State University, Ames, IA 50011-3171. (515) 294-5247, Fax: (515) 294-2945, E-Mail: pubdist@exnet.iastate.edu:

- "Cancer and Your Diet: Quiz" (1996)
- "Cholesterol in Your Body" (1996)
- "Family Nutrition Guide" (1997)
- "How to Eat without Raising Your Cholesterol" (1996)
- "Vegetarian Diets" (1996)

Available from **National Institutes of Health, National Cancer Institute** at (800) 4-CANCER:

- "Action Guide for Healthy Eating" (1997)
- "Eat 5 Fruits and Vegetables Every Day" (1997)
- "Tips on How to Eat Less Fat" (1997)
- "Time to Take Five: Eat 5 Fruits and Vegetables a Day" (1997)

Available from **United States Department of Agriculture**, Superintendent of Documents, U.S. Government Printing Office, Washington DC 20402 (202) 512-1800, Fax: (202) 512-2250, E-Mail: gpoaccess@gpo.gov, Internet: http://www.bookstore.gpo.gov/:

- "Team Nutrition's Food, Family and Fun: A Seasonal Guide to Healthy Eating: Commemorating 50 Years of School Lunch" (1996)

Available from the **University of Illinois, Cooperative Extension Services**, Ag. Publication Office, 67 Mumford Hall, University of Illinois, Urbana, IL 61801. (217) 333-2007, Internet: http://www.uiuc.edu/ccso/docs.html:

- "Food & Water: Partners for Survival" (1996)

- "Keeping Energy Levels Up" (1996)

- "Keeping Fluid Levels Up" (1997)

- "The Winning Connection: Sports & Nutrition" (1997)

Chapter 42

A Bibliography Of Cookbooks

There are literally thousands of cookbooks available. Some include recipes and instructions so simple a pre-schooler can follow along; some are for professional chefs; some focus on certain ingredients or themes; some are for people with special dietary concerns; some are for people who don't have time to cook; and some are for people who love spending a lot time in the kitchen.

The list included in this chapter is a small sample of the many, many cookbooks available. The books selected for inclusion were chosen because they had something to offer teens—features such as recipes for inexperienced chefs, recipes for people on the run, and tips on healthy eating habits. Inclusion does not constitute endorsement, however; and many fine cookbooks are not listed due to space constraints. If you have a favorite cookbook you'd like to suggest for inclusion in a future edition of this volume, please write to the editor at the address listed in the front pages of this book.

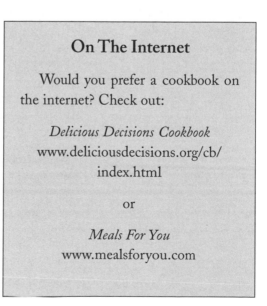

On The Internet

Would you prefer a cookbook on the internet? Check out:

Delicious Decisions Cookbook
www.deliciousdecisions.org/cb/
index.html

or

Meals For You
www.mealsforyou.com

The following cookbooks may be available at your local school or public library, or they may be purchased at a bookstore. They are listed alphabetically by title.

American Heart Association Low-Fat, Low Cholesterol Cookbook: Heart-Healthy, Easy-To-Make Recipes That Taste Great, by American Heart Association, Times Books, January 1998; ISBN: 0812926846.

American Heart Association Quick & Easy Cookbook: More Than 200 Healthful Recipes You Can Make in Minutes, by American Heart Association, Times Books, May 1998; ISBN: 0812930118.

American Medical Association Family Cookbook: Good Food That's Good for You, by Melanie Barnard, C. Wayne Callaway, Pocket Books, January 1999; ISBN: 0671536680.

Around the World Cookbook: Healthy Recipes With International Flavor, by American Heart Association, Times Books, November 1996; ISBN: 0812923448.

Better Homes and Gardens Low-Fat and Luscious: Breakfast, Snacks, Main Dishes, Side Dishes, Desserts, by Kristi Fuller (Editor), Meredith Books, February 1996; ISBN: 0696203731.

Betty Crocker's Good & Easy, by The Betty Crocker Editors, Macmillan Publishing Co. Inc., October 1997; ISBN: 002862288X.

Betty Crocker's New Low-Fat, Low-Cholesterol Cookbook, by The Betty Crocker Editors, IDG Books Worldwide, January 1996; ISBN: 0028603885.

Clueless in the Kitchen: A Cookbook for Teens, by Evelyn Raab, Firefly Books, March 1998; ISBN: 1552092240.

Cook Healthy Cook Quick, by The Oxmoor House Staff, Oxmoor House, Inc., February 1995; ISBN: 0848714245.

Cooking Light Five Star Recipes: The Best of 10 Years, by the *Cooking Light* editors, Leisure Arts, February 1997; ISBN: 0848715403.

Easy One-Dish Meals: Prevention Magazine's Quick & Healthy Low-Fat Cooking, by *Prevention Magazine* Health Book Editor, Rodale Press, Inc., September 1996; ISBN: 0875963250.

The Four Ingredient Cookbooks—Three Cookbooks in One! by Linda Coffee, Emily Cale, Cookbook Resources, September 1, 1998; ISBN: 0962855030.

Healthy Heart for Dummies/Lowfat Cooking for Dummies, by Lynn Fischer, IDG Books, January 2000; ISBN: 0764581376.

The Joy of Snacks: Good Nutrition for People Who Like to Snack, by Nancy Cooper, International Diabetes Center, April 1991; ISBN: 0937721824.

Moosewood Restaurant Low-Fat Favorites: Flavorful Recipes for Healthful Meals, by Pam Krauss (Editor), Clarkson Potter, November 1996; ISBN: 0517884941.

The New American Heart Association Cookbook: 25th Anniversary Edition, by American Heart Association, Times Books, January 1999; ISBN: 0812929543.

The New Classics Cookbook: Family Favorites Made Healthy for Today's Lifestyle, by Anne Egan, Rodale Press, October 1999; ISBN: 0875965032.

New Low-Fat Favorites: Fabulous Recipes from the World's Healthiest Cuisines, by Ruth A. Spear, Little Brown & Co., May 1998; ISBN: 0316806862.

Pillsbury Fast and Healthy Cookbook: 350 Easy Recipes for Everyday, by The Pillsbury Co., Clarkson Potter, April 1998; ISBN: 0609600850.

Quick & Healthy Recipes and Ideas: For People Who Say They Don't Have Time to Cook Healthy Meals by Brenda J. Ponichtera, Scaledown, September 1991; ISBN: 0962916005.

Quick & Healthy Volume II: More Help for People Who Say They Don't Have Time to Cook Healthy Meals, by Brenda J. Ponichtera, Scaledown, July 1995; ISBN: 0962916013.

Secrets of Fat-Free Italian Cooking: Over 200 Low-Fat and Fat-Free, Traditional & Contemporary Recipes—From Antipasto to Ziti, by Sandra Woodruff, Avery Publishing Group, October 1996; ISBN: 0895297485.

Silly Snacks, by Jennifer Darling (Editor), Better Homes and Gardens Books, September 1998; ISBN: 0696208474.

Simple Vegetarian Pleasures, by Jeanne Lemlin, HarperCollins, May 1998; ISBN: 006019135X.

Skinny Mexican Cooking, by Sue Spitler, Surrey Books, May 1996; ISBN: 0940625970.

The Teen's Vegetarian Cookbook, by Judy Krizmanic, Viking Press, May 1999; ISBN: 0140385061.

Vegetarian Express: Easy, Tasty, and Healthy Menus in 28 Minutes (Or Less), by Nava Atlas, Lillian Kayte, Little Brown & Co., June 1995; ISBN: 0316057401.

Vegetarian Soups for All Seasons: A Treasury of Bountiful Low-Fat Soups and Stews, Revised edition, by Nava Atlas, Little Brown & Co., October 1996; ISBN: 0316057339.

Weight Watchers: New Complete Cookbook, by The Weight Watchers editors, IDG Books Worldwide, January 2000; ISBN: 002863716X.

Index

Index

Page numbers that appear in *Italics* refer to illustrations. Page numbers that have a small 'n' after the page number refer to information shown as Notes at the beginning of each chapter. Page numbers that appear in **Bold** refer to information contained in boxes on that page (except Notes information at the beginning of each chapter).

A